T0384052

Routledge Revivals

The Unmasking of Medicine

Originally published in 1981 and then as a second edition, revised and updated in 1983 and now with a new Preface by Ian Kennedy, this is a hard-hitting and penetrating investigation behind the façade of late 20th Century medical thinking. Based on his controversial series of Reith Lectures, Ian Kennedy attacks issues and problems which are central to today's debate over the provision of health care. He asks why people are willing to give up so much power over their own lives to the medical profession and discusses why the Health Service has become an illness service. He also questions whether doctors are adequately trained to deal with ethical problems.

The Unmasking of Medicine

A Searching Look at Health Care Today

Ian Kennedy

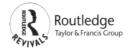

First published in Great Britain in 1981 by George Allen & Unwin Ltd. Published by Granada Publishing Limited in 1983.

This edition first published in 2023 by Routledge
4 Park Square, Milton Park, Abingdon, Oxon, OX14 4RN
and by Routledge
605 Third Avenue, New York, NY 10158

Routledge is an imprint of the Taylor & Francis Group, an informa business

ISBN 13: 978-1-032-65203-0 (hbk)
ISBN 13: 978-1-032-65207-8 (ebk)
ISBN 13: 978-1-032-65209-2 (pbk)
Book DOI 10.4324/9781032652078

IAN KENNEDY

The Unmasking of Medicine

A PALADIN BOOK

GRANADA
London Toronto Sydney New York

Published by Granada Publishing Limited in 1983

ISBN 0 586 08433 9

First published in Great Britain by
George Allen & Unwin Ltd 1981
Copyright © Ian Kennedy 1981, 1983
This edition has been revised by the author.

Granada Publishing Limited
Frogmore, St Albans, Herts AL2 2NF
and
36 Golden Square, London W1R 4AH
515 Madison Avenue, New York, NY 10022, USA
117 York Street, Sydney, NSW 2000, Australia
100 Skyway Avenue, Rexdale, Ontario, M9W 3A6, Canada
61 Beach Road, Auckland, New Zealand

Printed and bound in Great Britain by
Hazell Watson & Viney Ltd, Aylesbury
Set in Baskerville.

Granada®
Granada Publishing®

Contents

Preface

This book is an extended version of my 1980 Reith Lectures, entitled 'Unmasking Medicine'. Obviously the constraints of six half-hour lectures meant that I could not consider some points either at all or in much detail. So I have taken the opportunity to put a bit more flesh on the bones of my arguments and to add an extra chapter. I have also prepared a fairly extensive bibliography of sources, so as to help the reader whose appetite is whetted to find his way to other materials. This bibliography will also show how wide is the range of materials which someone venturing into this area of study needs to cover.

Perhaps I ought to identify the area. Fundamentally, it is the study of the practice of medicine today. In the United States the area goes by the name of 'Bioethics', a word I have never found terribly appealing. Here in the United Kingdom we do not seem to have a single label for it. Ethics and law together with sprinklings of philosophy, sociology and politics are all involved as they relate to medicine.

This is not a field in which it is necessary to be trained in medicine. Indeed, it could be said that it is only someone who is free from any claims which medical professional loyalty may make on his objectivity who can successfully examine the institution of medicine. I am a lawyer and have specialized in the field of medical law and ethics for some dozen years. Of course, a lawyer writing on medicine is, to some doctors, like a red rag to a bull. 'What about lawyers? Why don't you criticize them?' are questions I have frequently encountered. My only reply is that I happen to be interested in medicine. This does not mean that I think the legal profession is above examination and criticism, merely that such a task is for someone else.

Obviously, there are some issues, indeed many issues, which have not been dealt with in this book. The ones I have chosen reflect my view of what is important. Others might have made different choices. Furthermore, my choices reflect the need to paint with the broad brush, to explore certain general themes, since this is what I perceive to be the role of the Reith Lectures. It follows that I have tried to resist the temptation to pursue any question or matter in too much detail. This may upset some who look for a detailed treatment of, let us say, abortion, and do not find one. It seems to me that it would have been quite wrong to devote the Reith Lectures to the examination of a few individual topics in detail, although admittedly problems are tumbling over themselves for such consideration. Instead I decided it was appropriate to seek to explore and develop certain more general themes. This book reflects that choice.

Just as with the audience of the Reith Lectures, I would hope that readers will come from all sections of society. I have tried to avoid resort to technical language. It is for me virtually an article of faith that issues of great importance, touching on the way we live, ought to be aired and discussed as widely as possible. It is equally my strong conviction that there is no issue which is too complicated to be discussed before an interested and alert audience, provided it is presented in terms which are readily comprehensible. To argue otherwise is to surrender the power to decide to those who would claim the appropriate expertise, and thus to surrender part of that which is one's citizenship. Of course, it is for others to judge whether I have succeeded in these aims. I can only say that the reception my lectures have so far received has encouraged me to believe that I did reach a wide audience and that, whether they agreed with me or not, the large majority enjoyed the opportunity to explore these issues.

I chose as my title 'Unmasking Medicine'. My purpose is to ask some questions about the way medicine is thought of and practised, and to offer some ways of responding to what I perceive as problems. Clearly, reference to a mask suggests that a face is being presented which hides the real one. My aim is to expose and then examine the real face of medicine. To change the image, I am suggesting that medicine has developed its myths. My task is to dispel the myths, so as to discover what the truth may be. You will notice that I speak of the real face of medicine. It is the institution of medicine which I am examining. Clearly this means that I must look closely at the role doctors play, since it is around them that much of medicine revolves. Some will take this as just another case of 'doctor-bashing', but I hope that on mature reflection they will see my goal as something larger and more worthwhile than that. Indeed, I venture to suggest that, although there is criticism, there is also much that could be of help to doctors, if accepted and acted upon. For one theme I pursue is the need for each person to take greater responsibility for his own life, which includes his health. This can only serve to reduce the burden of responsibility now placed on doctors. I am quite sure we lay people do doctors a disservice by shuffling off on to them a range of problems which they should not be expected to deal with.

I do not intend here to offer some abbreviated version of what I say in the book. But let me offer some signposts. I am concerned with a number of themes. One is that of power — the power of the professional, here the doctor. I contrast with this power the notion of the self-determination of the client, the patient, and his sense of responsibility for himself. Another theme is that of the accountability of the doctor. I argue that there is a need to ensure that the decisions of doctors, to the extent that they are not technical, conform to principles acceptable to all of us. Admittedly, in a pluralist society there may not be any consensus, particularly on such troubling issues as abortion. But this is no reason why, even in such cases, the extent of the range of choices which are tolerable to the society at large should not be identified. Once identified, the doctors should then be expected to operate within them. A further theme is that medicine is, at bottom, a political enterprise. The choices we make as a society about how we govern ourselves, the values we espouse, dictate the kind of health we have, the kind of medical care we make available. Thus, if we are to improve our health, change our medical care, it is to government, not to doctors, that we must address our arguments. If such factors as poverty, malnutrition, stress, unemployment, and lack of job satisfaction are heavily implicated in undermining our health, it is clear these are not matters which doctors can affect.

Some, particularly the practical among you, will want to know what remedies I suggest, what plan of action I propose. You may well be disappointed that I seem to identify problems, ask questions, but do not offer too many answers. I could reply that it is a task in itself just to seek out the problems and ask the right questions. But I do not rest on this. Instead, my explanation is that I offer a particular view and seek to provoke a debate. If my view is rejected as being inaccurate or otherwise flawed, then so be it. Solutions will not be called for. If, as a consequence of debate, my view or something like it is deemed to be valid, then will be the time for the pursuit of answers, which will grow out of the debate. I offer some leads which may help. I suggest that we aim for a different destination. But I do not dwell greatly on the means of getting there, whether, metaphorically, it should be by train or by car or on foot. I see my role as a catalyst. I suppose I am that most irritating of persons – the one who believes that through discussion and education change for the better will emerge. Call it Utopian if you will. But, if you do, I feel you underestimate the power of ideas.

To some this book will be unpalatable. Certainly, it is aggressive in style and some may say that this is counter-productive in one who hopes to persuade. Well, that is a matter of judgement and I have made mine. I am fully aware that there are doctors who will dismiss (and some already have!) what I have to say as 'ludicrous' (*Medical News*, 1 January 1981) or an 'ill-conducted public rant' (*On Call*, 11 December 1980). This is hardly a surprise. There will always be minds which are closed. Some doctors will feel threatened. That is only natural. Others will say (and some have) that they have heard much of it before. This is, of course, no criticism; since if something is worth saying, it is worth repeating. But they should recall that I am not speaking only, or even primarily, to them. I am seeking to carry the debate out of the hushed halls of Academe into the noisy marketplace of ideas. I also like to think, if I may change my metaphor, that, although I have used red and green and yellow and a canvas just like others, the landscape I have painted is not the same as the one painted by the others, either in conception or in detail. I must, at the same time, of course, recognize those writers who have gone before, to whom my debt is great. Illich, McKeown, Muir Gray and Doyal come immediately to mind.

I have no illusions about changing society. I merely add my voice to that of others. Any changes which take place will, and must, come slowly, allowing all of us to adjust. At the same time, I offer this book to provoke some and to stimulate others. I also offer it as encouragement to those who cleave to the values we claim we stand for, a society which respects self-determination, within a context of democratic decision making, and which believes in the pursuit of health and a medical service free at time of use, with equality of access and care.

Let me finally make a couple of points concerning style and organization. The style throughout is that which I regarded as appropriate for a spoken lecture. I have not changed it. What it lacks in formality is compensated for in its directness. The fact that each lecture was part of a series and yet had to stand alone meant that there was inevitably some overlap of ideas. I have not sought to weed these out. Indeed, in the final additional chapter you will see that I return to several themes already touched upon so as to have the opportunity to consider them more closely. I could, of course, have done so by reworking the original lecture. But, I decided against this. It seemed to me that it would upset whatever overall structure and balance the lectures have.

It would be wrong of me to end this brief preface without thanking those who have helped me. A Research Fellowship from the British Academy helped me to finance much of my early research. My praise and respect for David Paterson, who produced the lectures for the BBC, cannot be overstated. He is the best of friends. He is a professional, and he is one of the most outstandingly able men I know. The faults in these lectures are mine. Much of the credit is his. George Fischer, Head of the BBC Radio Talks and Documentaries Department, offered me constant support. Peter Leek, my publisher, was suitably patient and a friendly guide. My brothers, Stuart and Alan, tolerated my long conversations and demolished many a bad idea. Andrea Gage looked after me and made it all possible.

IAN KENNEDY

Introduction to the Paladin edition

In preparing this revised edition, I had a number of aims in mind. I wanted to take account of some of the developments which have taken place in what is a wide-ranging and fast-moving subject; I wanted to argue some points more fully or more clearly; and, in certain contexts, I wanted to go beyond the point of posing questions, and offer for consideration some ways of resolving or dealing with them.

My original premise remains the same. It was, and is, to write a book about medicine; what it means for us, what it can and cannot do for us, how it is practised. I repeat what I said before – that it is not a book about the medical profession, far less is it an exercise in 'doctor-bashing'. There is a distinction between medicine and the medical profession, just as there is between architecture and architects, or law and lawyers. That consideration of medicine involves reference to the medical profession is obvious, but medical practitioners are only part of the story, as I seek to show particularly in Chapter 3.

Equally, I have tried to keep in mind the general reader, as well as the specialist. On a number of occasions in this revised edition I have chased down points of detail which previously I omitted. In so doing, I realize I run the risk of lapsing into too great a use of jargon or of over-complicating the point I am making. My hope is that the balance is about right.

It is fair to say that the reception which the book received from some reviewers when it first appeared was not ecstatic. Indeed, reading some reviews which friends (?) kindly sent to me, I was put in mind of a book review I once read in an American legal periodical which began, 'This is not a bad book. It is a very bad book!' I had, of course, expected some adverse comment. The public utterances from certain quarters which greeted the broadcasts of the Reith Lectures had prepared me. But I was still rather taken aback by the vehemence of the hostility of some reviews. One explanation may lie in the fact that editors of newspapers and journals tended to commission reviews from doctors in teaching hospitals, or psychiatrists, or medical scientists. Several of these never recovered from a first impression of feeling attacked, and by someone who was an academic and a lawyer. So they decided to teach me a lesson. The result was that there was much refutation by epithet, or by wrenching ideas or statements out of context. Reasoned argument tended to be the loser. An example of this genre, rather more moderate than most, and a response from me, can be found in some of the papers commissioned for the *Journal of Medical Ethics,* of December 1981. I welcomed and tried to learn from the comments of, for example, Sir Douglas Black in the *Journal* and elsewhere. But other remarks ranged from the hurt and wounded – 'I'm still proud to be a doctor, Mr Kennedy' of Professor Wilkes, again in the *Journal* – to the wonderfully, almost heroically, intemperate blasts from J.F. Watkins, in *The Times Literary Supplement* of 26 June 1981. While Watkins was not always anxious to engage in rational argument, it was clear he was having fun, as his closing words indicate: 'Unfortunately the public will assume that an invitation to deliver the Reith Lectures is a guarantee of respectability and importance – we may disagree with the lecturer's views, but they deserve to be heard. Surely the BBC would not allow the Reith Lectures to be devoted to trivia? On the contrary. An institution which runs a television comedy series about the SS is capable of anything.'

My strong feeling is that the sense of anger felt by some is now passing. Indeed, I have been immensely gratified by the response I have received from doctors and non-doctors alike, as I have travelled around debating and discussing. Indeed, the considerable volume of letters and comments I have received from many doctors as well as other members of the public was in some contrast to the reception I have just described. By and large, there was interest in, and often support for, the views advanced. And there was a general expression of relief that topics as important as the ones raised were being discussed in a form accessible to most who had the necessary interest. I do not say this out of any sense of self-justification, but rather to suggest that, not for the first time, those who would see themselves as guardians of medicine and spokesmen for the medical profession were profoundly out of touch with those they claim to speak for. I wonder sometimes how many times, for example, these people have visited post-graduate training sessions for GPs recently, and listened and contributed, as I have, as issues troubling to us all are discussed, not with rancour or hostility, but with genuine concern. I think it is probably true that the major, largely unstated, objection to my views which motivated these keepers of medicine's conscience was, and remains, what they perceive to be my political values. Some reviewers have gone out of their way to describe me or my ideas as 'populist' or 'egalitarian' (as if these were bad) or 'anti-authority' (and me a lawyer!). If proof were needed that medicine is, above all, a political enterprise, you have it here.

As I have said, I have tried to refer to some of the developments which have taken place since the book first appeared. The most striking is the great increase in public concern about and debate on the themes I touch on. Another has been the considerable upsurge of interest among medical students and young doctors in the teaching and study of medical ethics. It may well be a case of *post hoc, ergo propter hoc,* but I think some of this interest is a consequence of the Reith Lectures and this book. Equally, a number of multi-disciplinary committees have been set up recently to consider ethical issues in medical practice. Though I would prefer, as I argue in Chapter 4, the creation of a Permanent Standing Advisory Committee, something like the Law Commission, to keep under review ethical problems in medicine, these committees are a step in the right direction. Another area in which the pace of progress may have quickened is that of the detention and treatment of the mentally ill. Unfortunately, the Mental Health (Amendment) Bill is still winding its way through Parliament, so I have only been able to consider it in outline, as it is, of course, still subject to change as the appropriate compromises are struck.

There are many specific changes I have tried to take account of, such as the introduction of laws requiring the compulsory wearing of seat-belts, changes in the sick-note procedure, and shifts in governmental attitudes to the tobacco industry. Another is the increased interest in health education and health promotion, to the extent that recent meetings on these themes, bringing together professionals from a number of fields of health care, have been filled to overflowing in several parts of the country, whereas, as little as five years ago, they would have been poorly attended, if held at all. There has also been a number of court cases, the best-known of which is, perhaps, the trial of Dr Arthur on a charge of the murder, reduced subsequently to the attempted murder, of a three-day-old baby boy with Down's Syndrome. This and other cases attracted much public attention and provoked considerable discussion and debate, not all of it productive but, on the whole I think, worthwhile — all part of the process of dragging issues out of their dark corners and debating them in public which is a mark of a society's health.

These developments are the principal reason why this revised edition amounts virtually to a new book. I have rewritten Chapter 3 completely, made considerable changes and additions in Chapters 1 and 4 and at the end of Chapter 5, and minor changes throughout. There are also other reasons. I have tried to eliminate what I see and accept as a lack of clarity or inconsistency in my arguments, in particular in Chapter 1. The thesis has not changed, but I have sought to make it clearer. I have also emphasized more strongly than previously the difference between the medical model of health, which would have it that health is the product of medical care, and the social model, in which health is understood as the product of social, political and economic forces. I am not sure that I focused on this difference sufficiently in the previous edition. Finally, I have tried to go beyond the point at which I previously stopped. I specifically avoided offering proposals which might help to resolve some of the questions I raised because, at the time I was then writing, the degree of public interest and debate was not as great as it has since become. Open discussion is now almost a commonplace, thus I feel it incumbent on me to offer some more concrete proposals, to take the issues further, and I have done so where I think it may help.

This edition is now several stages removed from the original Reith Lectures. I have nonetheless tried to retain the style and form I used in the Lectures and in the first edition. The aim was immediacy of communication. At the same time, I have incorporated both minor changes and whole new sections. It may well be that this has strained the style, flow and continuity beyond what they ought to be asked to bear. I hope not.

Finally, I am happy to record my thanks to the Editors of *New Society* and the *Journal of the Royal College of Surgeons of Edinburgh* for allowing me to quote extensively from papers I wrote which first appeared in their Journals.

Preface to the Reissue – 40 Years on

For Gore Vidal, the 4 most beautiful words in the English language are 'I told you so'. Over 40 years ago, I offered my views on the state of medicine, first as the BBC's Reith Lectures, then as this book. You may think that little has changed.

The title *The Unmasking of Medicine*[1] invited my audience to see a world previously closed to most of them. With a greater democratisation of information, the expansion of education and entry into professions, and the explosion of the internet and social media, no unmasking is necessary. This world is entirely familiar.

Today's title would be: *Caring about Health and Healthcare*. My central concern was that these two are distinct. They need to be addressed separately. The neglect of health, not just what is called public health, but all those 'health affecting' forces I describe in Chapter 3, has grown worse. "Nanny state-ism" has seen off the pro-health forces. Regulation is anathematised, bequeathing us such legacies as an explosion in obesity, particularly in the young. The government's appallingly chaotic response to COVID 19 epitomised its neglect of the nation's welfare, leading to so much misery and death. As for healthcare, a government since 2010 committed to an ideology of 'small state' and shrinking support for and investment in public services has led to the increasing lack of healthcare professionals: we don't have enough and those we have are being ground down and leaving in droves. The death wish called Brexit made things even worse, further denying us much-needed staff not just in healthcare but in social care also, the crucial but disastrously neglected partner in caring for the frail.

---

1 A nervous BBC insisted on *Umasking Medicine* as the title of the broadcasts in case my view might be thought to be definitive!

Meanwhile, the National *Health* Service morphs ever more into what I describe in Chapters 2 and 3 as an 'illness service'. The balance between providing for health and responding to illness was wrong 40 years ago. It is much worse now.

In Chapter 3, I express particular concern at the health and welfare of children. 30 years later the Department of Health asked me to examine how children and young people fared in the NHS. 'Badly' was my conclusion. I warned of an 'epidemic' of mental health problems. 13 years on, except for the privileged few, things are even worse. In addition to inequalities in access to education, healthy nutrition and leisure activities, the lives of the next generation are blighted by a new addiction - the screens on their phones; their brains rewired, their minds routed down rabbit holes where they confront the worst imaginings of the Inferno, persuaded of their inadequacies – in body shape, looks, or friendliness. Faced with this burgeoning social disaster, government does what government has done for so long – nothing. In bed with the corporate class, enjoying the donations, lauding the values of 'free speech' pushed by the Zuckerbergs of the world, they may make the occasional speech expressing concern – but otherwise, nothing.

Chapter 4 on ethics caused the greatest stir. Many doctors felt challenged, as if I were intruding in their world. But quite quickly my view that ethics was for all of us gained acceptance. Medical Schools, regulators and Royal Colleges invited ethics in. This is to be welcomed. There's a danger, however, that doctors' and nurses' exposure is only skin deep – philosophy lives in the world of norms and 'oughts', a world unfamiliar to those used to science and evidence. The paradox is that you have an awareness of the importance of ethics without a real

grasp of how to do it. Take one example. When I chaired the Bristol Inquiry, we heard a young doctor talk of 'consenting' a patient. I was non-plussed. Doctors don't 'consent' patients, I interjected, they ask for consent. Yet this is what the young doctor had been taught. The whole relationship between patient and doctor is turned on its head. The doctor takes control in the very circumstance in which control belongs to the patient. 20 years on I frequently encounter patients being 'consented'. Skin deep ethics is almost as dangerous as no ethics.

You may find my treatment of mental health in Chapter 5 odd. At the time, I was concerned with the elusive nature of the concept of mental illness. The argument is still worth having, not least as regards the reach and consequences of the label. This led to my concern for the civil liberties of those assessed as mentally ill. Although these concerns remain, the law, at least in theory, now offers greater protection. Now my concerns are twofold: first, the growing incidence of what now are described as mental health problems because of the policy of 'austerity', a.k.a. the steady hollowing out of public services, alongside unemployment, homelessness and a widespread sense of despair at the growing inequality people see around them. Second, there is the shameful lack of care available to the growing number of those who need help. The services are not there. The specialists are not there. The NHS is not there. The only thing that is there is the growing line of people who are left to suffer, often taking refuge in street drugs because they cannot get care. The elderly in particular continue to suffer the twin ills of isolation and loneliness.

Chapter 6 has 2 themes which remain dear to my heart. The first is clinical negligence litigation. It should have been abolished 40 years ago. It remains with us. It is unfinished business. I appeared before a House of Commons Committee in November 2021 to make my case again. The Committee accepted it. They agreed that patients harmed by healthcare should receive appropriate financial and medical support, paid from general taxation. They should not have to sue, nor even to identify what caused the harm. *Separately*, there should be an investigation into what happened, informed by human factors analysis. Lessons should be learned and disseminated. Any failings in performance should be addressed and dealt with by employers and regulators. Sadly, though unsurprisingly, the Committee's Report has been ignored. The current bill for outstanding legal claims is £83billion and rising. It's madness.

The second theme is regulation. I hinted at it in calling for an inspectorate. 25 years later the first regulator of the NHS was created with me as Chair. It was a start. The model based on measuring performance against data which I introduced[2] was soon replaced by

2 See my essay *Learning from Bristol: Are We?*

one relying more on visits/inspections – the traditional regulatory model which I regard as flawed. Moreover, the regulator was positioned more as police force than promoter of improvement. These are unfortunate developments, but regulation is still unfamiliar to the NHS (as well as poison to the free marketeers on the current government benches) and viewed with suspicion. I hope that over time the data-based model designed in 2006 will regain favour.

There were 6 Reith Lectures. Chapter 7 was extra. Let me just add a word about technology. The last 40 years have seen remarkable developments. The next decades will be no different. I have high hopes for the deployment of AI, for example, in the early identification of illness. CRISPR and stem cell research will bring significant benefits. But it is important that ethical analysis goes hand in hand. The recent reports of the creation of an artificial embryo should be welcomed if it allows for better understanding of early development but should remind us to be alert to ethical challenges.

As I write, a challenge of a different, existential kind looms, a challenge to the very notion of the vision of a Welfare State imagined by Beveridge and implemented by the Atlee government. Talk is everywhere of the need for 'structural change,' a new 'model'. This is code, not seriously disguised, for abandoning 'care free at the point of need' funded from general taxation in favour of some sort of insurance based system, a system from which money can be made.

I argued several months ago[3] that the past decade and a half had witnessed the slow, intentional undermining of the NHS, to reach a point when the call for an alternative would be too deafening to ignore.

It should be ignored. In my submission to the Times Health Commission in June 2023, I urged the retention of Beveridge's vision: '… the state should make appropriate arrangements for the health and healthcare of its citizens through general taxation, as being the fairest way of funding provided the taxation system itself is rendered suitably fair – addressing, for example, tax avoidance schemes, off-shore operations and, critically, focussing on wealth as well as income as a source of revenue). Those who reject this conclusion must show

3 *New European*, Dec 8, 2022

that any alternative will be the equal of or better than the Beveridge
model or offer a different vision of society in which matters such as
fairness and equality of access to the enjoyment of society's goods
are less important than other goals.'

You may feel that this new preface is too gloomy and even angry.
There is much to be gloomy and angry about when surveying the
state of the nation's health and healthcare.

Make it change!

Ian Kennedy, July 2023.

Other writing

Learning From Bristol, Department of Health. 2001
https://assets.publishing.service.gov.uk/government/uploads/system/uploads/at-
tachment_data/file/273320/5363.pdf
Learning from Bristol: Are We? Healthcare Commission, 2008 ISBN: 1-84562-
10402
https://assets.publishing.service.gov.uk/government/uploads/system/uploads/at-
tachment_data/file/273320/5363.pdf
Getting it right for children and young persons, Department of Health. 2010 https://
assets.publishing.service.gov.uk/government/uploads/system/uploads/attach-
ment_data/file/216282/dh_119446.pdf
Kennedy Review – Paterson's Breast Cancer Surgery, Heartlands NHS Foundation Trust.
2013 https://hgs.uhb.nhs.uk/wp-content/uploads/Kennedy-Report-Final.pdf
Healthcare Law and Ethics: Selected Essays, Hart. 2021 https://www.bloomsbury-
collections.com/book/healthcare-law-and-ethics-and-the-challenges-of-public-
policy-making-selected-essays/index
Clinical Negligence Litigation, Prospect. December 2021
NHS Dream or Nightmare, New European. December 8, 2022 https://www.the-
neweuropean.co.uk/the-nhs-dream-is-dying/
Thoughts on Health and Healthcare – Submission to the Times Health Commission.
(as yet unpublished in June 2023).

1   The rhetoric of medicine

Six years ago, the American Psychiatric Association took a vote and decided homosexuality was not an illness. So, since 1974 – at least to the APA – it has not been an illness. How extraordinary, you may think, to decide what illness is by taking a vote. What exactly is going on here?

I have set as my task the unmasking of medicine. It is not that I think there is something sinister behind the mask. But I do detect a sense of curiosity, of concern if not disquiet. The practice of medicine has changed. There is a feeling abroad that all may not be well. This feeling grows out of a sense of distance, out of a sense that medicine is in the hands of experts and sets its own path. *We* can take it or leave it. Heart transplants, the definition of death, the treatment of the dying, the sad fate of Karen Quinlan, the selective treatment of handicapped newly-born babies, the treatment of the mentally ill – there is a long list of issues which are deeply troubling but which seem effectively to be kept under wraps. One of the most successful ways of doing this is by making the issues and problems appear to be medical, technical ones, not really for the rest of us at all. This can be accomplished by the simple device of translating the issue into medical language. I do not mean by this translating it into the technical terms we associate with medicine, but embracing it within the conceptual framework of medicine. The first step on the way to *understanding* modern medicine, looking behind the mask, is to unravel the *rhetoric* of medicine.

Let me begin with the word 'illness'. It is, you say, a word you understand. You know what it means and it will take more than one curious example from the activities of the American Psychiatric Association to persuade you otherwise. 'Illness', you insist, is a technical term, a term of scientific exactitude. Whether someone has an illness, is ill, is a matter of objective fact.

But homosexuality is as much a part of social life after 1974 as it was before. The objective facts have not changed. What has changed is how the particular doctors choose to judge it. This suggests the strangely disquieting insight that illness involves not merely the existence of certain facts. It involves a judgement on those facts. And it is doctors who do the judging. A choice exists whether to categorize particular circumstances as amounting to an illness. Power is vested in the doctor, and the power is not insignificant.

It becomes important, then, to discover whether there are boundaries to this word, this concept 'illness'. Can it be applied willy-nilly, on the say-so of the doctor, or are there limits to his power? To analyse the word 'illness' is to explore the role of the doctor in modern medicine. It is to discover that medical practice is above all a political enterprise, one in which judgements about the proper order and governance of society are made.

But, you ask, are there not *many* conditions about which we would all agree that they constitute illnesses. Of course, the answer is yes, there are. Obviously we all agree that someone with an inflamed appendix is ill, as is someone who cannot breathe very well, even when resting. Equally, we agree that someone with, say, leprosy or cancer is ill. Why do we all agree? It is obvious, you say. Someone with an inflamed appendix *is* ill. He has got appendicitis. But this is a circular argument. We have to go more carefully. What we have is certain facts about the physical condition of a person. We all agree that these are illnesses because we accept two propositions. The first is that there is a normal state in which the appendix is not inflamed and breathing is easy while resting. Second, it is appropriate to judge someone who deviates from this norm as ill. Only if we examine both of these will we understand what is involved in the meaning of the word 'illness'.

Take the first of the two propositions, that there must be a deviation from the normal state. This seems simple enough. It is not, of course. For a start, it is our convention to call such deviations from the norm illnesses. But let it be clear that there is no logical necessity to call a set of physical symptoms an illness. Others, in other cultures, may view such conditions entirely differently. They may see them as visitations from the gods, as punishments deserved and to be accepted, or as possession by spirits. We cleave to science and the scientific principle of a demonstrable state of normality and a causative agent which brings about an abnormality. Few would object to this convention. Even so, we still have a problem. What is the state we should regard as normal?

A common method of answering this is to have recourse to an analogy drawn from engineering. We think in terms of a machine which has a design, which is the norm, and which malfunctions when it does not perform according to the design. Indeed, in common speech we may describe our car as sick, or ill, or on its last legs. And, by and large, this analogy serves us well. But it has its shortcomings. One weakness is that it is crude. We like to think of ourselves as more than machines. We have emotions, moods and feelings which affect profoundly our physical state. A further weakness is that we may not all agree on the design, the blueprint, against which to measure our performance or our state. For example, women have the capacity to bear children. In the old days, it was considered part of the design for women that they bore children. A woman who did not bear children departed from this design. She was to that extent abnormal. She was described as barren, a term with connotations of illness as well as some notion of moral judgement upon her. You will recall that Julius Caesar urged his wife to touch Antony so as to be cured of her barrenness.

To some extent we have changed our view of the design for women. There is probably less inclination now to attach to childless women a term suggesting illness or moral judgement. The point, however, is clear. The normal state, against which to measure abnormality, is a product of social and cultural values and expectations. It is not some static, objectively identifiable fact. As views and values change, so the norm will change. So, if illness has as its first criterion some deviation from the norm, some abnormality, it too will vary and change in its meaning.

And the influence of social and cultural values does not stop there. The meaning of illness is subject to the values we bring to bear not only in deciding what is abnormal, but also in how we ought to judge this abnormality. Take, for example, the tension and interplay which has always existed between illness and evil. It is a commonplace that at different times the same abnormality may be viewed as illness or evil. Before the days of modern medicine it was common to regard conditions we now regard as illnesses as being attributable to possession by evil spirits. For example, some of those accused of witchcraft by Cotton Mather in seventeenth-century Massachusetts would probably now be described as epileptics or suffering from Huntington's chorea, a fatal congenital illness characterized by uncontrollable shaking and gradual mental degeneration. They would now be seen as ill, and certainly not as evil.

The notion of possession has, however, retained some of its vitality. The old idea that particular states were caused by devils or demons possessing the sufferer fell before the onslaught of scientific medicine. But scientific medicine has not abandoned the notion of possession. Indeed, it is as strong as ever. What has changed is the identification of the possessing force. Demons become germs, spirits become diseases.

Equally, we have fluctuated in our views as to whether the user of certain drugs or the alcoholic is ill or evil. The user of morphine and later heroin was regarded in the late nineteenth century as someone perhaps deserving of sympathy because of his dependence on 'medication'. He was, however, still someone worthy of respect or a position of authority. Estimates suggest that between 2 and 3 per cent of the United States' population were habituated and dependent upon opiates at the end of the nineteenth century. Such a proportion in the United States now would be about eight times the number of present-day users of heroin. Within twenty years a change of enormous significance had taken place. Users were no longer looked on so benignly. The view had emerged that they should be divided into the ill and the evil. Troy Duster, in his book *The Legislation of Morality*, cites an article by G. Swaine in 1918 in the *American Journal of Clinical Medicine* in which users were divided into two classes.

'In class one', Swaine wrote, 'we can include all of the physical, mental and moral defectives, the tramps, hoboes, idlers, loaders, irresponsibles, criminals and denizens of the underworld . . . In these cases, morphine addiction is a vice, as well as a disorder resulting from narcotic poisoning. These are the "drug fiends". In class two, we have many types of good citizens who have become addicted to the use of the drug innocently and who are in every sense of the word, "victims". Morphine is no respecter of persons, and the victims are doctors, lawyers, ministers, artists, actors, judges, congressmen, senators, priests, authors, women, girls, all of whom realize their condition and want to be cured. In these cases, morphine-addiction is not a vice, but an incubus, and, when they are cured, they stay cured.'

What had happened was that in 1914 the Harrison Narcotic Act had been passed. A crucial provision was that a user could obtain his heroin or morphine only on a doctor's prescription. In 1919 the Supreme Court of the United States, in *Webb* v. *US*, considered what was the effect of the provision in the Act that a prescription could be given only for 'legitimate medical purposes'. The Court decided that 'a prescription of drugs for an addict, not in the course of professional treatment in the attempted cure of the habit, but being issued for the purpose of providing the user with morphine sufficient to keep him comfortable by maintaining his customary use was not a prescription in the meaning of the law and was not included within the exemption for the doctor-patient relationship'.

The habituated user, cut off from a lawful supply, had to go underground, to the criminal black market. The climate was created for what Duster calls 'a moral reassessment of what had previously been regarded as a physiological problem'. Opiate users could be reclassified as criminals and therefore morally evil. The motive for the Harrison Act was well-meaning paternalism, to protect an unsuspecting population from the habituating qualities of opiates. The result, however, was to allow, and thereby cause, drug use to be seen in moral terms, and the user to be judged evil, if he otherwise qualified for social disapprobation.

Furthermore, at any one time, we may be ambivalent in how we judge some particular abnormality, whether as illness or as evil, or indeed, whether as illness but also having some quality of evil. There is, in many contexts, a subtle relation between ill and evil whereby the description 'ill' can carry with it a marked undertone of moral judgement and condemnation. When we describe someone as ill, we often say that he has got something wrong with him. And it is important to notice that the word 'wrong' can also connote lack of moral worth. Furthermore, an illness often takes on a metaphorical quality whereby it becomes a condemnation of some social ill. Something is a cancer in our midst or is pestilential. Or a person may be said to be ill − as is, for example, the alcoholic − but in the next breath it may be said that he has only got himself to blame, or he is very weak, where weak is synonymous with lack of moral strength.

Running through all these examples is, of course, the central theme of responsibility. As our views of each person's power to exercise dominion over his life change, so will our concept of the borders between illness and evil. Evil is deemed to be a product of a person's choice and therefore something for which he is responsible. Illness, by contrast, is something which overtakes him. Once ill, he is absolved from the ordinary responsibilities of everyday life.

So illness, a central concept of medicine, is not a matter of objective scientific fact. Instead, it is a term used to describe deviation from a notional norm. So, a choice exists whether to call someone ill. The choice depends upon the norm chosen and this is a matter of social and political judgement. As the great American scholar Oliver Wendell Holmes remarked, at the end of the nineteenth century, 'the truth is that medicine, professedly founded on observation, is as sensitive to outside influences, political, religious, philosophical, imaginative, as is the barometer to the changes of atmospheric density'. Ordinarily there will be widespread agreement about what objective facts, what physical states are appropriately described as abnormal. But this does not belie the fact that there is an inherent vagueness in the term 'illness'. And this is only the beginning. Even when it has been decided that the physical conditions warrant the description 'abnormal', there is still the second step. They have to be *judged* to be illness. An evaluation has to take place.

This should cause us to pause. Who does the evaluating? What are the values involved? Does this mean that the vagueness we previously noticed is compounded? Does this mean that the concept of illness can be put to different uses, that it has no clear and certain boundaries? We began with the cosy assumption that illness was a descriptive term, applied to a set of objective facts. It appears now that illness is an indeterminate concept, the product of social, political and moral values, which, as we have seen, fluctuate. The implications of this will strike you immediately. If illness is a judgement, the practice of medicine can be understood in terms of power. He who makes the judgement wields the power.

Let me explain what follows from this. The treatment of illness is for doctors. A social institution has grown up defined and managed by doctors, the role of which is to persuade us that our preoccupations must be related to them, and them alone (since they alone have competence). We appear, perforce, naked both physically and emotionally. However willing we may be, and however well intentioned the doctor, it is hard to overstate the power which this vests in the doctor. It is hard to overstate how such a social arrangement may undermine the notion of individual responsibility and of course, ultimately, individual liberty.

Michel Foucault, the contemporary French philosopher, captures the point perfectly, as Richard Sennett made clear in his review in the *New Yorker* of Foucault's most recent book, *The History of Sexuality*. Foucault, writes Sennett, argues that 'in the modern world all too often there is no clear line between concern for the welfare of others and coercive control of their lives'. 'A new kind of power relationship has arisen in modern society,' he goes on. 'Authorities who understand our bodies have gained the right to make and enforce rules about morality.' The nature of the power relationship is seen in terms of confession, now to medical rather than priestly 'authorities'. In the past the person who confessed furnished the raw data, the confessor the meaning, and so it is today, according to Foucault.

Interpretation and with it judgement and prescription become the preserve of authority, since, knowing what we do not know about ourselves, doctors acquire the right to show us how to behave. Let me take this further. So far, I have mentioned only the interplay between illness and morality. A far more significant interplay exists on a political and social plane. Just because illness is associated with objective facts, it appears that illness *is* those facts, that illness is a thing. But, as we have seen, illness is not a thing, it is a judgemental term. Being ill is not a state, it is a status, to be granted or withheld by those who have the power to do so. Status connotes a particular position in society, assumed only after satisfying others that certain conditions have been observed. In the context of illness, it is the doctor who must be satisfied. Illness, then, has become a technical term in that, in its proper sense, it is for doctors to use. Others, of course, may and do use the word, but they use it by analogy to real illness, which is the province of the doctor.

Let me explain. Consider Mr Brown. He is an old man who lives alone in an untidy flat. He has difficulty paying the rent; he has less and less money to spend on food and heating. A neighbour one day arranges for a doctor to visit him. The facts are clear — he is cold and hungry. But is he ill? Does he qualify for the status ill? If he is said to be ill he may qualify for certain additional social welfare benefits. He may also use his new status as a bargaining counter in persuading his children to visit him. On the other hand, if he is ill, he may have to go into hospital. If this happens, he is likely to lose his flat and have nowhere to go, except some form of institutionalized home. And, if he is ill, he may lose his independence, which he has prized so much, and become reliant upon others. The doctor's judgement that he is ill would lend legitimacy to his claims, but set in motion the events he fears.

The doctor may take one of several views. He may decide that Mr Brown is a cantankerous old man who deserves his fate and for whom he can do nothing. Such a judgment would, of course, be expressed in terms suggesting that there is nothing the matter with Mr Brown. The exercise of power in denying the status ill lies hidden in this apparent description. On the other hand, the doctor may decide that Mr Brown needs some help, but not from a doctor. He will then contact the various social welfare agencies and advise them that although Mr Brown is not ill, he does need assistance. In this way the doctor serves to confer the status on Mr Brown, not of being ill, but of being a recipient of welfare. This may well be the last thing Mr Brown wants, since he resents, in his old-fashioned way, the stigma he attaches to welfare. And his children will be able to argue not only that he is not ill, but also that he is being looked after, to the extent that they need not concern themselves.

The doctor may, however, decide that Mr Brown is ill. The facts concerning Mr Brown are constant. The judgements vary. They vary according to the values the doctor brings to bear in judging those facts. They vary depending upon how the doctor wishes to exercise his power. They vary according to the use to which the doctor chooses to put the word illness. Locked within them are complex matters which go unnoticed and unanalysed − for example, the doctor's views on the values or otherwise of independence, on the obligations of family members to each other, on the usefulness of the social welfare services, on the legitimacy of assigning Mr Brown's case to these services which are charges on the taxpayer's purse, on the relative merits of the Samaritan or the Levite in our society, on the consequences for the health service, or for Mr Brown, of diagnosing him as ill.

Let me offer another example. Consider Mr Smith. He works on an assembly line. He finds the work dull and tedious. One day, he decides he has had enough and would like just a few days at home. Until 14 June 1982, he presented himself to his doctor and asked for a certificate, excusing him from work. Let us analyse this process carefully. The first stage is the understanding by Smith that he needs authoritative affirmation that he is ill. He may decide he is ill. Indeed it is a feature of modern medicine that, outside emergencies, it is the individual who makes the first decision concerning illness. He stakes a claim to illness. But his decision is not enough. The monopoly power to confirm or deny the presence of illness rests with the doctor. Notice I used the word power, not skill, since it is more than a technical power. The doctor may say, 'Yes, Mr Smith, you ought to have a few days off', and then add a diagnostic tag such as stress or overwork (overwork being clearly an evaluative term). Smith then gets his certificate. Or the doctor may say, 'There is nothing the matter with you, Smith.' His notes may read, 'Another malingerer'.

What process is involved here? What sort of term is 'malingering'? It involves a judgement that Smith ought to be working and that the doctor is not going to aid him in receiving benefits while avoiding this responsibility. Another doctor could just as well decide otherwise. Besides the power the doctor has to manipulate the concept of illness according to his view of what is socially or politically proper, several other points emerge from this example. One is that a major use of the term 'illness' is in a functional sense. Is the person able to function in the role he has? Consider the power this gives the doctor. He may have no idea of what life on an assembly line is like, yet he has the power to decide whether Smith should get back to it or not.

Second, it suggests that one of the functions most clearly involved in the notion of illness is the capacity to work, at least as regards adult males. Health comes to be defined as the ability to work. Of course, this is no new thing. The great public health reforms of the nineteenth century were motivated more by economic than humanitarian considerations. As Henry Chadwick wrote, 'Of all those who are born of labouring classes in Manchester more than 57 per cent die before they attain 5 years of age, that is, before they can be engaged in factory labour.'

Third, it follows from this that Smith the complainer is not seen as a unique individual with unique needs but rather as a unit in an economic system. The doctor reflects and enforces certain political values. Productivity is expected of labour. Rest is a reward to be earned.

Fourth, there exists always the opportunity to exercise class bias in the ascription of illness. The blue-collar worker may be conceived of in terms which demand that, whether through brutishness or fortitude, he be less susceptible to stress while the white-collar worker is deemed, probably quite wrongly, to be exposed to greater stress and to warrant more sympathy and tolerance. After all, he works with his brain — an argument which ignores the proposition that mindless work may by its very mindlessness be that much more stressful. There are, of course, numerous other examples of class bias in the manipulation of the concept of illness. For example, consider what happened behind the trenches during the First World War. The private who offered the excuse of shell-shock to explain his wandering off or his refusal to obey orders ran the risk of being shot. The officer was classified LMF, 'lacking moral fibre', and was shipped back to

Britain. Victorian ladies of the middle class were seen as victims of their bodies, prone to nervous emotions and needing to rest. This view did not, however, extend to those women working long hours in the factories or the mills.

I choose the example of the sickness certificate for Mr Smith not because it suits my purpose but because it has, for so long, been so common and so clear. The conclusion exists that illness is a spurious scientific term and that the doctor in purporting to determine its existence as an objective fact is engaged in a series of moral, social and political choices which we permit him to make.

It must be said that many doctors found the position they were put in most unsavoury. Frequent protests led the Department of Health to change the form of the sickness note in 1976. Eventually, as I indicated, the system was considerably altered, with effect from June 1982. Under this new system, a worker who wishes to obtain sickness benefit may certify himself as unfit for work, provided that the period away from work is less than seven days. The new scheme represents, if you will, an explicit recognition of the fact that the doctor's decision whether or not to give a worker a sick note put the doctor in the invidious position of having to make what was, in effect, a judgment of a social and political nature.

The fact that the worker now certifies himself as unfit for work, however, could be said to contradict my view that illness is a technical term uniquely within the province of doctors. I do not think it does. All it does is to recognize that a worker may wish to be absent from work, and that he may be allowed to get away with it for a few days (sickness benefit from the State is not paid until the fourth consecutive day of absence from work), leaving it to the employer, in the true traditions of market forces, to control this. It is a realistic acceptance of the facts of life. In turn, it saves doctors a lot of time otherwise spent certifying illness for workers. But a closer examination of the rest of the scheme suggests that my thesis is intact, for several reasons. First, if he wishes to be absent from work for more than seven days, the worker still needs a doctor's certificate. In other words, if he is saying that he is 'really' ill, he must submit himself to a doctor. Only in this way may the status of ill be legitimately acquired. Secondly, a number of company schemes which provide for sickness benefit require a doctor's certificate after three or four days, just like the old system, before benefit will be paid. It is likely that this requirement will become more common. And, of course, it represents the employer's view that while a worker may say he is unfit for work for the purposes of the State's social security benefits, he will only get their benefits if he is again 'really' ill. Furthermore, the doctor is recruited to achieve this end, and will be able to charge a fee for this extra service.

Thirdly, under the new scheme, a worker who has certified himself as unfit on four occasions in a year, will have his records sent to the regional medical officer and will, on a fifth application for benefit, be required to submit himself to a doctor for examination. He will, in other words, have to prove, once again, that he is 'really' ill. Only a doctor, it is assumed, can demonstrate this. And, most interestingly, as *The Times* of 14 June 1982 reports, on this fifth occasion, 'the claim for benefit would be considered in the light of the report of the regional medical officer *and the past history of claims*' (my emphasis). Thus, in sum, the point I make concerning the power of the doctor in this context remains valid, though in a somewhat altered form.

The basic system remains and with it the power. The doctor is engaged in a process of socialization, of ensuring that certain social and political attitudes and values are reinforced and are adhered to by those who, by their behaviour, may be seen as potential deviants. For, as Muir Gray puts it, 'deviance is not a property inherent in certain forms of behaviour: it is a property conferred upon these forms by the audience which witnesses them'.

If you remain unconvinced of the view I am advancing, consider Mrs Jones. Married at nineteen, she is now thirty-five. She stays at home all day, while her husband is at work and their children are at school. She has grown to dread and despise the tedium of her life. She finds her husband boring. She feels trapped. She has ambivalent emotions towards her children. Life, she feels, is passing her by. She finds herself crying most days. She decides to visit her doctor. She has diagnosed herself as needing help and chosen the doctor in the absence of other obvious candidates as the appropriate provider. She may not think of herself as ill. Indeed, in previous times she may have consulted her priest although not thinking of herself as sinful or in danger of perdition. Her doctor tells her that she is anxious and depressed, something she already knew. The doctor can then confer on her the status of ill, if he so chooses, by offering to treat her through the use of his medical expertise. He will provide antidepressants or tranquillizers. More than two-thirds of all prescriptions for such drugs are for women rather than men. It may be no coincidence that women appear fifteen times more frequently than men in advertisements addressed to doctors for mood-changing drugs.

What does this commerce between the two of them signify? The doctor is prepared to use the flexible term 'illness' to embrace Mrs Jones's condition. By so doing, he endows himself with power over her and satisfies his own and her desire that something be done. A further implication is that he affirms that Mrs Jones is ill, because is not he treating her? He affirms that her condition is abnormal and that medical intervention is therefore warranted to bring her back to normal. Other women cope. Coping is good. Coping is the norm. But Mrs Jones's complaint is her dissatisfaction with a social and economic order which robs her of independence and ties her to her home. The doctor cannot change the economic and social order, but, with drugs, he can stop her worrying about it. So that is what he does. He returns her to the ranks of unhappy women who no longer feel the pain. By so doing, of course, he prevents the rancour she feels from being expressed in political or social terms. The social and economic *status quo* is maintained, through the agency of the doctor. He becomes, once again, an agent of a particular form of social system ensuring that its values persist.

This is not to say that the doctor's role is sinister or conspiratorial. In some large part the doctor acts as a socializer quite unwittingly. His education has trained him to see illness and to try to ease pain, even if by so doing he merely drives the cork deeper into the bottle, so making uncorking that much more explosive. The doctor is not, of course, wholly unaware, though he may be disquieted. He may know what he is doing. He must resort to such arguments as, 'Should I just let her go on being unhappy? That would be too cruel.' It is a hard question to decide which course is the more cruel. Recently a Liverpool doctor, many of whose patients are now unemployed, described on BBC radio how they came to him for 'a Vali', a Valium tablet. He said he really did not know what to do. He could not give them a job. They were clearly anxious and depressed, yet he was reluctant to prescribe drugs for something he saw as a political ill.

I do not say that the doctor should not prescribe the Valium for Mrs Jones or for the unemployed Liverpudlian. I deliberately refrain here from expressing a view because, at this juncture, I am seeking only to make the point that the doctor has to decide, and, in so doing, is inevitably involved in the exercise of power. That such decisions are excruciatingly difficult, I do not dispute for a moment. They call for the most careful analysis of the role of the doctor in society and his duty to the patient, both as a patient and as a member of a group. These issues are sufficiently complex to warrant more than a passing reference here, and I shall return to them later in some detail in my discussion of medical ethics. I am, at this stage, doing no more than seeking to establish what cannot be a difficult proposition to accept, namely that doctors, like all professionals, have power. This is a social reality. They have knowledge and skills; their clients do not, and are supplicants. The question, surely, is not whether doctors have power, but how it is used and whose interests it should serve.

It is fair to say, however, that my references to power offend or disturb some doctors. Dr Michael Thomas, Chairman of the British Medical Association's Central Ethical Committee, writes in the *Journal of Medical Ethics* of December 1981 that my view 'implies that doctors have aggregated power to themselves as part of a plan of aggrandizement'. I venture to suggest that he misunderstands my argument. He, with others, would give to the word power a pejorative connotation. But this is quite wrong. Power is an abstract property. It can be used for good or ill. My concern is that the ability of clients to affect their relationship with professional advisers, such as doctors, is directly related to the power which the professional is able to assert, asserts, and is allowed to assert, and the values reflected in this process. As Jonsen, Siegler and Winslade argue, in their useful book *Clinical Ethics*, 'physicians have enormous power in these [physician-patient] relationships. They can shape the course and the moral dimensions of medical care by their psychological dominance, specialized knowledge, and technical skills. The physician's power can, if misused, undermine the therapeutic relationship and destroy the fragile moral autonomy of the patient.' If the desired end of all professional-client relationships is a relationship of mutual trust and responsibility, power cannot and should not rest with the professional alone, nor should the values reflected be those of the professional alone, or of a particular section of the community whose interests coincide.

Of course, we, the public, have connived at the ways in which doctors have exercised this power. We have avoided responsibility, content to let others decide for us, whatever the decision, whether out of ignorance, or trust, or — interestingly — even out of choice. We may well seek sometimes the childlike irresponsibility that illness endows upon us. There is nothing like being ill occasionally. You are waited on hand and foot, excused from responsibility, indulged and pampered. How many of us have pleaded 'Doctor's orders', when explaining why we cannot perform some particularly tiresome social duty? Victorian ladies avoided all sorts of crises by an attack of vapours and a call for the doctor, and a headache has been a godsend to many an embattled female. As Susan Sontag argues in her book *Illness as Metaphor*, nineteenth-century Romantics developed the idea of invalidism as a pretext for leisure and an escape from bourgeois responsibilities. It was 'a way of retiring from the world without having to take responsibility for the decision'. We have opted on occasions for what Illich has called the medicalization of life, the conversion of social and political ills into illnesses.

Some of you may say that I have given an exaggerated account, that there is a lack of balance here. Well, the examples of Mr Brown, Mr Smith and Mrs Jones, so far from being unusual, are among the most common encounters between doctors and patients. Indeed, just to mention Mrs Jones, it should be noticed that close to 10 per cent of all prescriptions written by general practitioners are for tranquillizers, antidepressants, or hypnotic drugs, at an annual cost of about one-fifth of the annual expenditure of the NHS on drugs.

If further evidence is called for, consider the following. To demonstrate, first, the evaluative element implicit in the notion of illness, take someone who had difficulty in breathing as a child. He can be told that there is nothing the matter with him that cannot be avoided by a few simple precautions or he can be told that he is ill, that he has asthma. To choose the latter course is to label him and to cause him to think of himself as an invalid for the rest of his life. From someone who cannot run, he becomes someone who should not run. To illustrate, secondly, the way in which illness is determined by reference to social factors, take, for example, the medicalization of bereavement. Someone who is grieving is now deemed to be in need of medical care and, perhaps, drugs. Or again, consider a girl who has a bad bite or crooked teeth. She is told that her teeth need to be corrected. Her condition which warrants medical intervention is that she deviates from a socially determined ideal of beauty. Anyone who does not meet this ideal has something wrong with her. Or again, scratchy throats, runny noses, or headaches can be converted into illnesses and the growth of the speciality of allergy treatment has indeed brought this about. Or again, a study in South Wales, as David Robinson in his book *The Process of Becoming Ill* reports, showed how tiredness was taken for granted as a normal state of everyday life by members of the working class but was likely to be seen as a sign of illness by those in the middle class. Another example may be the growth of certain mass screening procedures. These have sometimes had the unfortunate consequence of persuading people who felt perfectly well beforehand that they are 'susceptible', or 'at risk', or in a 'pre-whatever-it-is state', thereby causing them to think of themselves thereafter as ill, even though nothing is different. Perhaps the supreme example of this epidemic of illness lies in the area of mental illness. I shall consider this at much greater length later. Suffice it to say here that the categories of mental illness seem never to be closed and that candidates for the status 'ill' are constantly emerging to fill the categories developed by those whose interest lies in the continuation of this process, those who specialize in mental illness.

Let me now move to a further point. There is within the concept of illness a further element. We tend to confine the use of the word to certain circumstances. We demand of the aspirant to the status 'ill' the condition that he be capable of getting better, of recovering from his illness. Illness is regarded as a transient state bounded by optimism. Notice that we tend not to use the term in a number of situations despite the fact that there is a clear deviation from the notion of an objective physiological norm. For example, we do not describe those who have lost a limb, or gone blind, or deaf, as ill. We may use the word 'invalid' or 'disabled' but not 'ill'. In using these other terms we reveal once again the close relationship between the language we use and the values of our society. *In*valid has the same root as in*va*lid, like a bad cheque. It does not work, it has no force, it has no worth. The change in pronunciation helps us to hide the harshness of this judgement and its reflection of the values of production and economic worth. Disabled is only slightly less harsh. The person so described is no longer able, he cannot do, and one adds the words, anything or anything much. Again the values of an industrial, production-oriented society emerge.

Take now the terms 'chronically ill' and 'terminally ill'. As regards chronically ill, there is no optimism here, so the adverb 'chronically' is used to signal the fact that this is not ordinary illness, but a special status with its own special rules. The same is true of 'terminally ill'. This term is a product of the modern obsession with death. Clearly, someone who is dying will not recover. Yet our pathetic search for immortality has led us to think of dying as an illness, because, by so categorizing it, we hope, perhaps magically, to introduce a note of optimism, a remote possibility of getting better. But rationally we realize that we must separate it from the general status of ill, so again we use the qualifying adverb 'terminally'. Thus, we are true to reason without abandoning irrational hopes! A final example is the term 'handicapped'. Once again this connotes someone who is less than competitive in the market and thereby again reflects societal views of life as being rooted in economic values.

Why do I dwell on this? Circumstances have been marked off in which the term 'illness' is not 'properly' to be used, or is to be used only with qualification. It is no coincidence that these are areas in which the doctor's power to do anything is much limited. The term 'illness' has become reserved 'properly' for circumstances in which recovery is possible, or, at least, treatment, intervention can be justified. Thus the doctor gratifies himself in his adopted role as healer, a role identified for him in medical school, and retains his status and credibility with the public, by conditioning his power and claim to competence by reference to the chances of success. This is not to say that doctors cannot do much for the chronically ill or disabled. They both can and do. It is only to say that the separate categorization of such people serves as a signal that what can properly be expected of the doctor is different. A further unfortunate consequence of this process is that persons consigned to a status other than ill 'properly so-called' may be less well thought of and certainly less well cared for. Doctors, for the most part, will opt out of devoting themselves to people who offer no obvious reward, no prospect of achieving something by way of cure. This is perhaps one important but overlooked reason why the handicapped, the chronically ill and the disabled are so severely neglected in our society. The terminally ill may be the exception, because, while it is true that most languish in unhappiness buoyed only by the devotion of nurses, the growth of the societal preoccupation with death has persuaded doctors to enter this field as merchants of hope, at least of temporary respite, through surgery, chemotherapy and the like.

In conclusion, I am not saying that we should abandon the use of the word 'illness'. I am merely urging that we understand what it involves. Since the diagnosis of illness always calls for a judgment, it is right for us all to consider when it is properly to be applied and who should set the ground rules for its application. We should consider what limits may properly be placed by us on the power of doctors to manipulate the concept. I am not suggesting that we take a vote. But we must make it our business to ensure that the judgements arrived at reflect the considered views of all of us. Each diagnosis of illness is an ethical decision.

So far I have concentrated on the term 'illness'. Let me now consider the concept of health. Health, if it is to have any useful meaning, must refer to more than the mere absence of illness. It must have a positive quality. For example, a man who, for want of anything else to do, lies in bed all day may not have any illness, may in that sense be well, but would not ordinarily be described as leading a healthy life. Health must refer to all those factors which combine to represent man's aspirations and expectations. But, if expressed in this way, once again you see at once that here is no term of nice exactitude. It is in short an evaluative term, redolent with moral, spiritual, political and social overtones and by no means limited to bodily functioning. This is captured in the World Health Organization's definition of health as 'not the mere absence of disease, but total physical, mental and social well-being'. This definition, however, so far from serving as a blueprint for planning and policy, whether for governments or doctors, is often held up for ridicule, even by doctors.

'What is the use of this sort of airy-fairy thinking?' the argument goes. 'We cannot do anything about these things. We have got enough on our hands dealing with the illness about us. We cannot make people richer or more comfortable or whatever total well-being means.'

But let us consider this ridicule for a moment. To embrace a notion of health which calls for positive political action and the creation of appropriate economic and social conditions is to concede that 'health' is fundamentally a political term. This most doctors are unwilling to do. They see themselves and want to be seen as scientists, not the political and social agents I have suggested they often are. And to adopt this approach would be to call for some movement away from investing the greater part of our resources in attempting to remedy existing illness (a never-ending exercise), towards the principle of preventing, checking or controlling, through social and political action, many of the conditions which give rise to illness. Very many of the people to whom we are readily prepared to ascribe the status 'ill' find themselves ill because they are poor, grow up in bad housing, eat poor food, work, if at all, at depressing jobs, and generally exist on the margin of survival. The doctor, because of the way medicine has developed, sees himself as powerless in these matters, except as a voting citizen along with everyone else. And his professional vote goes to retaining a notion of health tied to illness, because here he is all-powerful. The doctor is the entrepreneur of illness. Quite contrary to the view of Sir James Bryce, that 'medicine is the only profession that labours incessantly to destroy the reason for its own existence', the opposite is true. We have abdicated to doctors the power to define health, with the result that it is predominantly defined in terms of illness and disease. We have all come, quite wrongly, to think of health only in these terms. We have come to think that medicine holds the key to health. And as long as it is accepted that health is the exclusive preserve of doctors, something only they have competence in, this state of affairs will continue. It is a matter of balance. The power now is with the professional. Only when it is realized that health is far too important to be left entirely to doctors, that it is a matter for all of us, will conditions be created for the necessary redirection of effort and resources. Only then will any real movement towards health be achieved.

Let me end my examination of the rhetoric of medicine by considering the word 'disease'. Disease has become a central concept of medicine. It has brought in its wake a number of unfortunate consequences. Dr Bernard Dixon remarks in an article in *Omni* of July 1980 that although there may be some slow rethinking of this concept it still wields tremendous force, such that 'orthodox medicine is strait-jacketed by it'.

Let me explain. If illness involves, at least in part, an abnormal condition, then this abnormality is thought of in terms of a disease. Immediately you will notice the danger, at least intellectually, of this approach. We have seen that illness is not a thing, but a judgement. Nonetheless, preoccupation with disease has meant that we have misled ourselves into thinking of illness in essentialist terms, as having a specific essence, of being a thing. Illness becomes the occupation (or possession) of the body by an entity called a disease, caused by some particular agent. You will notice an earlier religious precursor of this approach, the possession of the body by spirits, a view which still prevails in certain parts of the world. There is a further impeccable pedigree in the case of Pandora, sent as a punishment by Zeus, complete with her box, containing as Robert Graves puts it 'all the spites that might plague mankind'. The great spites or plagues of the previous centuries, which brought illness and death, were infections, such as cholera, TB, diphtheria, typhoid, typhus, smallpox, whooping cough and scarlet fever. TB accounted for 17.6 per cent of all the deaths in the first Report of the Registrar-General in 1839 and the real figure may have been closer to one-third of all deaths. There was little understanding of how these infections operated, what caused them to break out and how to survive them.

The idea that infection could be caused by germs was developed in the late nineteenth century. These infections are memories now, at least in the United Kingdom and other rich industrialized countries. Contrary to popular view, it was not modern medicine which caused them to disappear. Their disappearance, as Professor Thomas McKeown so clearly demonstrates in his book· *The Role of Medicine*, was due, overwhelmingly, to three factors: improved housing and sanitation, improved nutrition, and improved methods of birth control whereby demands on food and physical resources were reduced. By the time that prophylactic measures were available against them, these infections had in fact all but disappeared as major threats, at least in terms of bringing widespread death or serious disablement. This is not to overlook the enormous value of vaccination and immunization in ensuring that pockets of infection do not break out from time to time.

There is no doubt that the disappearance of the threat from the major infections has been a magnificent boon. But in terms of the development of modern medicine it has had two unfortunate consequences. The first is that the elimination of the major infections has served as the basic evidence, the star witness if you will, of the triumph of modern medicine over illness. A mythology has emerged with metaphors of battle, triumph, conquest: the patient's defences are threatened, the tumour is bombarded after invading the body. The doctor is categorized as the crusader constantly called upon to wage a holy war upon the enemy called disease, in some way a third party distinct from doctor or patient. And not only is the doctor fighting a war; it is also part of the mythology, based on the elimination of infectious diseases, that he will win. Disease will be vanquished. Life will be sweet. Of course, when examined calmly, the basis of the claim is suspect. Just as infections in the nineteenth century were not conquered by medicine, so much of today's illness seems curiously resistant to medical attention. Nonetheless, it is thought churlish if not downright treasonous to doubt the story or ask too many questions.

The other unfortunate consequence of the elimination of major infections is that it has provided the intellectual basis for the development and refinement of the notion of disease, as it is now understood. What we now think of as disease is some specific entity, which is caused by an attack on or invasion of a part or parts of the body, or by some malfunction of a part, so as to produce circumstances in which someone complains of feeling ill. The idea has grown up of a one-to-one relationship between disease and its causative agent. The idea of specific aetiology grows out of this, although first suggested by Thomas Sydenham in the seventeenth century. Admittedly, as Toon writes in the *Journal of Medical Ethics* of December 1981, 'the use of the terms "disease" and "diseases" has come under increasing scrutiny in recent years'. He argues that, 'Medicine is leaving behind the idea . . . of "specific diseases caused by specific agents", if indeed it was ever held'. It would be a mistake, however, to equate his efforts and those of a few other philosophically-oriented medical scientists to develop a new and rationally more defensible theory of disease with a whole intellectual shift within medicine. Such a shift is nowhere in sight. Any new thinking is to be welcomed if it will lead to an escape from essentialism. But the fact remains that the classic disease theory I have described still conditions the thinking of doctors and, through them, of the public at large.

From evil spirit to germ to infection to disease entity, we have seen attempts to reify or personify a something which once identified can be dealt with. The impact of scientific thinking has provided the ideal climate for this development. The earlier Hippocratic tradition of concern for the whole person in his environment, which had its practical worth in guaranteeing that Greek colonies were established in healthy places, has been ousted by the post-Renaissance view that illness is a mechanical failure. The Cartesian notion of the body as a machine has remained a central thesis. Like the machine, the body has functioning parts, each of which, with proper taxonomical skill, skill in classifying, has to be listed and its function explained. And, just as the machine will not run for long if a fan-belt breaks or a gear cog is stripped, so your body will not function properly if, for example, your kidneys malfunction or are attacked. Humans have been reduced through the application of impeccable scientific skills to ambulatory assemblages of parts. Just as medical scientists have identified and tagged the parts of the body, they have persuaded themselves that they can identify and tag those things called diseases. We have witnessed a great flowering in taxonomy whereby genus, species and sub-species of disease have been set down.

Two observations are in order. First, intellectually satisfying as it may be to develop this taxonomy, it is of little use unless it leads to being able to do anything. Often medical care begins and ends with diagnosis. Second, and far more serious, disease theory has led to an attitude whereby the malady is seen as somehow separate from the sufferer. The disease is what has to be treated, not the person. But we are more than a set of functioning parts. To regard us as such, as machines, is to overlook the great complexity of each of us. It overlooks the subtle interdependence and interrelationship of the parts which make up the whole. For example, in a paper published in the *New England Journal of Medicine* in December 1979, Vaillant reported on a study of the health of 204 men over four decades. He demonstrates clearly that the physical health of the subjects in mid-life was significantly related to their state of mental well-being, as illustrated by such indicators as job satisfaction, job promotion, recreation with others, marital stability and holidays.

What is wrong with the concept of disease is not that there is no malfunctioning part. There may be. Rather, it is that medicine has come to concentrate on it to the exclusion of all else. Disease theory has induced a sort of medical tunnel vision. What is not seen, as one critic puts it, is the sick person in all his wholeness and variability. Of course, there are doctors who do try to treat the person rather than just the disease. To them what I am saying may appear unwarranted criticism. I would reply by saying that the mentality of treating the disease is widespread and deeply entrenched. Second, given the estimated average contact time between GP and patient of between five and six minutes, the possibilities for treating the person are slim. In other words, the institutional framework within which medicine is practised militates against such an approach.

Furthermore, it is clearly bad science to conceive of illness in terms of specific diseases caused by specific agents. As René Dubos has pointed out, when Robert Koch announced his discovery of the tubercle bacillus he should have realized that all in the room must have been exposed to it in their lifetime, yet they had not suffered from TB. Thus the bacillus was only part of the story. Nutrition, fatigue and other environmental factors were as important in converting something harmless to some into something deadly to many. In Ecuador, for example, the World Bank reports that measles has a mortality rate 247 times higher than in the United States.

But this alleged scientific approach receives constant reinforcement from two principal sources. First, it is socially and intellectually gratifying for doctors to think of themselves and be thought of as scientists. It connotes working in the realm of knowledge and truth, light years away from the barber and the bleeder of the past. It carries a desirable social cachet. Furthermore, it allows for specialization and sub-specialization in tune with the taxonomical categorization of diseases. This allows doctors to mark themselves off from each other, and by creating the supply they provoke the demand. Diseases follow the categories, not vice versa, and, of course, specialization carries its own risks for the patient. As one wag has put it, surgery is often like killing a fly on a window-pane with a hammer. You kill the fly, but also smash the window. 'But', he went on, 'if you have a hammer in your hand, everything starts to look like a nail.'

The second source of reinforcement for the notion of disease comes from those who have a vested interest in the continued vitality of the notion of specific disease entities. I think particularly of the pharmaceutical industry. The relation between the manufacturers of pharmaceutical products, medical education and, consequently, how medicine is thought of and practised, warrants careful attention. In the middle of the nineteenth century it was discovered that by-products of coal and later of petroleum refinement could be used to manufacture synthetic dyes, chemicals and drugs. Production of pharmaceutical products grew in conjunction with the development of the petroleum and petrochemical industry. If doctors could be persuaded to reorient medicine towards the notion of pharmaco-therapy, then, clearly, here were riches indeed. Enterprises such as the Rockefeller organization began to pour some of their wealth into educational foundations. The major interest of these foundations was medicine. In 1910, Abraham Flexner, a professional educator, produced in the United States his famous report on medical education commissioned by the Carnegie Foundation. He recommended a shift to science-based, professionalized education which would exclude other approaches to medicine, thereafter stigmatized as quackery. Pharmacology was to be an integral part of the curriculum. The approach to health was to be interventionist, including the use, not surprisingly, of drugs. Thereafter medical education was massively funded by foundations whose money came from petro-chemical and pharmaceutical products. Rockefeller wealth was the largest single private source of capital for medical science and education. Eli Lilly, the drug company, has spent $250 million on medical schools in the United States over the past fifty years or so. The aim, as the Director of Research of a Congressional Committee put it, was to produce a curriculum designed to indoctrinate the student, particularly in the use of drugs.

An early worker in the field, Paul Erlich, coined the term 'the magic bullet' to describe Salvarsan, the drug which was developed around 1910 to treat syphilis. The metaphor of the bullet is of course intended. The disease existed as a specific entity and would by the application of the drug be eliminated. One unfortunate feature of the metaphor, which is with us more and more now, is, of course, that bullets are only as good as the aim with which they are fired. Furthermore, they tend often to fail to discriminate between the intended target and other things behind, in front, and round about. But the image has been enormously successful, so that modern medicine is now almost totally preoccupied with disease identification and disease-specific response, 'symptom-swatting', as one writer has put it. In effect, of course, there are occasions in which recourse to drugs more closely resembles writing the name of your intended victim on a bomb and then throwing it into a crowded restaurant where he is eating. Indeed, the term 'side-effect' has had to be coined to designate 'unwanted' effects. An effect is an effect for all its being called a side-effect. This is an obvious case of sleight of hand.

This is not to say of course that all pharmacological intervention is misconceived. This would be stupid, in the light of such magnificent developments as the sulphonomides and the antibiotics. It is to say that it has helped to produce or reinforce an attitude to illness which is wrong-headed. First, by concentrating on disease, a form of medicine has developed which, besides being mechanical, is conceived of as a rescue or repair service. You wait metaphorically until the car does not work and then you seek to make it work by squirting oil at it or changing some part. Second, the major infections have gone, largely without the help of medicine, and analogies or analyses based upon them are unhelpful. It seems clear that the traditional response of disease identification and disease-specific intervention has made little impact on the incidence of the present ills we endure, though it has undoubtedly made some easier to endure. Third, to concentrate on illness in the form of disease-entities diminishes us both spiritually and physically. Illness, feeling ill and wanting assistance, implies a process far more complicated and subtle than the metaphorical replacement of a fan-belt. Finally, it is wrong-headed in that, by thinking of illness in terms of disease, we have been led to believe that diagnosis leads to cure.

This, sadly, is far from accurate. There is little to be gained from labelling if not much can be done once the label has been arrived at. And, of course, the history of modern medicine in overall terms is that just as it was not responsible for the elimination of infections in the nineteenth and early twentieth centuries so it has had very little impact on the death rate since then. It has had considerable impact on the sickness rate from certain ills, but only limited success in the case of others, particularly those which are the most common amongst us, such as tooth decay, digestive disorder, skeletal and muscular disabilities, the common cold, heart ailments, coughs and bronchitis, accidents at work and home, stress, pain and un-happiness. But the myth persists. The whirligig of disease identifi-cation goes round and no one seems anxious to stop it or get off. I do not say we should not use the word 'disease'. I merely urge that we understand the dangers implicit in its use.

I have examined three of the central concepts of modern medicine. You have seen some of the implications they hold. They imply judgment and evaluations. If we are to take back power to control our lives, if we are to press, for example, for better health, if we are to ensure that illness does not become a substitute for unhappiness or being unwanted, we can and must understand and examine these judgments and evaluations. We must notice how they are applied. We must ensure they conform to our sense of what is right or appropriate. We, through the various mechanisms of our democratic society, must keep a watchful eye on what is done in the name of medicine. We must become the masters of medicine, not its servants. Let there be no misunderstanding: in the politics of medicine, it is we who must have the power, we who must set the policies. Educating ourselves in the language of medicine is the first step. Our next step is to look at the way modern medicine has developed — and examine how in many respects it has taken the wrong road.

2 The new magicians

My view can be stated briefly. Modern medicine has taken the wrong path. An inappropriate form of medicine has been created, in large part by doctors and medical scientists, and eagerly accepted by a willing populace. I will go further. The nature of modern medicine makes it positively deleterious to the health and well-being of the population. We have all been willing participants in allowing the creation of a myth, because it seems to serve our interests to believe that health can be achieved, illness can be vanquished and death postponed until further notice, while it serves the interests of doctors to see themselves and be seen as, if not miracle workers (and of course they would be the first to deny this), then at least possible miracle workers.

Science has destroyed our faith in religion. Reason has challenged our trust in magic. What more appropriate result could there be than the appearance of new magicians and priests wrapped in the cloak of science and reason? Please understand that it is we, all of us, who have hitched our wagon to the wrong star, scientific medicine. The unhappy consequence is that medicine is perceived and pursued in ways which do not best serve the needs of society. We do not put to best use the skills and abilities of those who have become its practitioners.

Let me explain in a series of points what I see as the path taken by modern medicine and how it may be the wrong one. I intend to concentrate on doctors and their attitudes and training. They may represent only 7 per cent of the National Health Service work-force, as against, for example, nurses, who represent 43 per cent, but it is they, the doctors, who spend the money and hold the power. The 1979 Report of the Royal Commission on the National Health Service, in the most comprehensive review of the Health Service since its creation in 1948, put it as follows, 'They [doctors] are responsible for initiating the expenditure in the National Health Service,' and 'play an important role in the management of the financial resources of the service.' Let me make it clear at the outset that what is involved here is a question of emphasis and balance. I know we can all point to many worthy features of medicine. But on balance I find modern medicine wanting.

At the outset, it is crucial for understanding that certain ground be cleared before the enquiry can proceed. Medicine has perhaps two primary goals. One is the maintenance and promotion of health. The other is the care and treatment of the sick. In the achievement of the first goal, that of health, medicine can play only a relatively minor role. We have seen already that health, properly understood, is the product of the complex interaction of political, economic and social forces, well beyond the power of those who work in the name of medicine to control. They include such diverse factors as the level of affluence we have, the food we eat, the home we live in and the job (if any) we have. For the most part, however, health is not perceived in these terms. The medical model of health, which has it that health is the product of medical care and the intervention of doctors, dominates the thinking of doctors. And we, of course, have also come to be persuaded to accept this view. This is not only unfortunate and misleading, it is calculated to produce attitudes and policies positively antithetical to producing and maintaining health. The social model of health, quite simply, is successfully elbowed out. It barely gets a look-in. As a consequence, we have been persuaded to look to medicine to provide us with health, rather than to ourselves, to Government and to our social and political institutions. This is the first sense in which medicine has taken the wrong path, and I make this point here because it is so important in establishing the background against which any discussion of medicine must take place. I will return to it again and again, here and subsequently.

There is also, here, a second sense in which we can talk of a wrong turn. For, even in those circumstances in which medicine can have any real effect on our health, the way in which it is conceived of, taught and practised takes it in directions which are not such as to achieve the results it is capable of, nor necessarily productive of health. If we turn to the second goal of medicine, caring for those whose health is impaired, here again, on balance, medicine has taken the wrong path. This is what, in particular, I want to suggest in the points which follow.

First, as now taught and practised, medicine is avowedly and self-consciously scientific. Far be it from me to stand against the tide of history and suggest there is more to understanding and caring than contained within the four corners of science. But an education which demands high skills in scientific subjects before going to medical school, and involves years of breathing the heady air of one field after another of scientific endeavour once there, produces what it is intended to produce: a doctor who sees himself as a scientist. It may not produce what is so often needed: someone who can care. I am not suggesting that medical education should not be scientific. Of course it must. But room must be found for other disciplines, particularly the humanities.

In his survey of medical education in 1978, *Quest for Excellence in Medical Education*, Sir George Pickering complained of the growing regimentation of the doctor in training, whereby the student is forced into an intellectual strait-jacket. Changes intended to cause doctors to address the social context of a patient's complaint and seek to involve the various social services have been made and this is now reflected somewhat in practice. But a fundamental problem remains, in that the doctor still sees himself as separate from these services, to which, at some point, he hands over his patients. As the 1979 Royal Commission on the NHS reported, 'Critics of the undergraduate medical curriculum argued to us that medical education was not well-adjusted to the working world, that . . . it produced a doctor whose skills, attitudes and expectations were sometimes poorly related to the health problems and needs of the community.'

The late Professor Henry Miller, who was Dean at Newcastle Medical School, wrote, in *Medicine and Society*, that much thought has gone into attempts to reshape medical education away from the old model of basic science followed by the plunge into clinical care. A greater attempt has been made to involve students with patients from the outset and most medical schools now devote some teaching time to courses which seek to relate medicine to the society in which it is practised. That said, he observed that the emphasis was still fundamentally scientific, such that the 'crisis in medical education still remained unsolved'. Pickering concluded that, 'for the vast majority of students in Great Britain, the medical curriculum is virtually as it was thirty years ago'. Moreover, the science now taught only compounds the problem. It is concerned with reaction, response to ills which already ail the sufferer. Far greater emphasis should be placed on inquiring into the causes and origins of illness, with a view to preventing them. So medicine may be called the healing art, but in the practice of that art it is the scientific method which is portrayed as the best, if not the only way.

My next point is that modern medicine has come to be thought of as dispensing cures. The image created of medicine has increasingly become that of a curative discipline in which the model of the doctor is that of the engineer/mechanic applying the techniques of medical science to cure a sick engine. This reaches its high point in what I see as an attitude to death in which dying has come to be regarded as an illness. Call it an illness and you hold out hope of treatment, control and even cure. Doctor, patient and family become locked in an unholy *danse macabre*. Medicine provides another variation on the theme of the pursuit of immortality, with the respirator symbolizing some kind of Promethean eternity. But the engineer/mechanic model is an unfortunate one. Quite simply, the problems that beset us now do not seem readily amenable to cure. And I speak now of the generality of ills: those that kill us before our time, such as cancer, heart disease, respiratory problems, and accidents; or those that chip away at our daily pursuit of tranquillity − colds and coughs, aches and pains and simple unhappiness. I do not seek, indeed it would be quite wrong, to belittle the contribution scientific medicine has made and continues to make, both in curing infections, at least in their short-term effects, and in controlling and soothing numerous otherwise intolerable conditions − in reducing sickness, even if it has had little effect on mortality.

But, as John Loraine points out in his recent book, *Global Signposts to the 21st Century*, 'the enthusiasm for engineering medicine contrasts vividly with the rather meagre advantages which have accrued·to health through its application'. This is so despite such extravagances as ex-President Nixon's 'war on cancer', declared in the National Cancer Act of 1971 and presumably still being fought, although annual deaths from cancer in the United States continue to rise, if only because cancer is predominantly a disease of the old, and, as the population gets older, so more die from it than from some other cause. The most common causes of death and the most common debilitating diseases still remain beyond the reach of the doctor. Cures there are not.

The idea of the doctor as an engineer, applying scientific principles directed towards cures, produces a further consequence, which I shall make my third point. It is that doctors are encouraged to adopt the mentality of problem-solvers. Problems exist out there in the world which it is their job to solve. What is wrong with that? Well, it is wrong in several respects. It is a mentality which creates problems. Indeed, the more efficiently doctors look for problems, the more they find and the more problem-solvers we need. It is a mentality which converts modern medical care into crisis care. We wait for a crisis, a problem, then we take it to the doctor and expect him to solve it. It is a mentality which fosters the impression that the problem can be solved, an impression all of us readily adopt. Finally, it is a mentality which ignores the notion that problems can be avoided, that waiting for them to arise and then responding to them is a less than adequate way of providing health care.

Fourth, another consequence of perceiving medicine as a scientific exercise has meant that it is conceptualized and practised largely in terms of specific diseases. Medicine is thus committed to a process of reductionism. The totality of a complex human being, the product of innumerable forces, involving subtle balances and interrelationships, is broken down. He becomes no more than a collection of parts, one or more of which is diseased. Each disease then has its particular name, *locus* and nature. It is this entity called the disease which then receives attention, not the person. As I said earlier, I am not suggesting that we should abandon the notion of disease. It serves a purpose and anyway it is too much a part of our vocabulary to exorcize it now. But, if illness is seen only in terms of specific diseases, this induces a form of tunnel vision. The very skill of the doctor with detail may cause him to lose sight of the whole. Miss A becomes an X-ray projected on a screen, Baby B becomes a bad case of meningitis, Mr C becomes the pain in the neck at four o'clock.

Of course, I readily concede that there are doctors who would regard this as an unwarranted criticism, who seek to practise a type of medicine which looks to all the circumstances of the patient. They are, I would suggest, adopting such an approach despite their formal training rather than as a consequence of it. They are responding to the reality of the problems they confront. Theirs are not as yet, however, the views and values which direct the future shape of medicine.

My fifth point is that modern medicine teaches that the appropriate response of the doctor to our complaint is to do something, and something aimed at a particular disease entity. If he has been educated to think of himself as an applied scientist and problem-solver and if there is a disease lurking somewhere, then it is his job to seek it out and remedy it. This has meant that medical responses have more and more taken the form of action against a disease entity, whether surgical excision, or irradiation, or chemical destruction or, if these are not possible, symptomatic relief. Whatever is decided upon, some form of bodily intervention which is disease-specific is usually sought. Something must be done to satisfy both the expectations of the patient and the professional pride of the doctor, and it has to be done to the disease, which is portrayed in terms redolent of morality or religion, as something bad, or wrong, which is possessing the body. The process has become one of applying taxonomical skills so as to identify the disease and then deciding upon the appropriate disease-specific response.

Indeed the process may be even less complicated. A study conducted by members of the Institute of Medical Sociology of the University of Aberdeen showed that the consultant, knowing the limited range of treatments he has available, is typically concerned from the outset of his contact with the patient with the simple question: 'Which treatment is most suitable?' The choice is then validated by appeal to the diagnosis.

What is wrong with this mentality of doing something? It is medicine by reflex: wait for the problem and do something. It causes larger and more important questions to be ignored, such as how the state of affairs came about, or what the long- or short-term effects of the chosen response will be. It is particularly unlikely that the question 'Should anything be done at all?' will be raised. These questions will tend to be lost in the display of pseudo-scientific wizardry.

The doctor is not alone in cultivating this mentality. You only have to look at advertisements in the press or on television to see how the notion of disease and disease-specific response is manipulated by drug companies so as to sell their products. Diagrams, effective for all their banality, show target areas with the product winging its way to knock out pain, indigestion, headache or whatever, and of course no one encourages this more than we ourselves. It is so much more satisfying to know that you have arthritis than to be unsure about what is the matter. The knowledge operates to put your mind at ease. It could, after all, have been another disease of greater menace on the

'Richter' scale. But such knowledge says nothing about whether the illness could have been avoided or what impact it will make on your future lifestyle.

The sixth point concerning the inappropriate form medicine has taken is that medicine is increasingly thought of in terms of hospitals. Indeed, the number of hospitals is often cited as a measure of the quality of health care. For example, as Michael Ryan points out in his book *The Organization of Soviet Medical Care*, the Soviet Union was able to claim in the mid-1970s that, except for Sweden and Norway, it had overtaken all other industrialized nations in the ratio of hospital beds to population size. The implication was that its system of health care had equally advanced, despite the long-standing inadequacy of its primary care services, particularly in the countryside. The nonsense of this approach is obvious. Indeed, apart from units concerned with accidents and, perhaps to a limited extent, obstetrics, the fact that an ever-increasing proportion of our Health Service budget, now around 65 per cent, goes to hospitals could be said to be evidence of the failures of health care and how we perceive it.

If ever there was a case of putting the cart before the horse, this is it. If preventive medicine, school health care, community health care and general primary care meant anything, hospitals would be far less needed. Hospitals are the epitome of the problem-solving, disease-oriented, applied science, engineering approach. And this idea of hospital-dominated medicine is constantly reinforced in our minds, if only by such things as radio and television programmes, whether they take the form of a soap-opera or a demonstration of the 'gee-whiz' surgical skills displayed in such BBC television programmes as 'Your Life in Their Hands'. In early 1982, for example, the BBC, in its wisdom, showed seven forty-minute-long documentaries devoted to telling all there is to be told, in the greatest detail, about heart transplants. The sublime technical skills involved in these operations and the gripping drama of the life and death struggle they represent, make them more attractive to the unthinking producer or journalist, anxious only for ratings, than the humdrum life of the health visitor or the occupational therapist. So, a particular and skewed image is presented of medical practice, which invites the conclusion of the man in the street that not only is this what medicine is, but it is also what medicine ought to be. And, of course, the present growth of private medical care, with its almost exclusive emphasis on hospitals and high revenue surgery, feeds successfully on this image.

The reasons why medicine is increasingly equated with hospitals are many. Medical students are trained in hospitals. Hospitals are where they learn to see themselves as applied scientists, problem-solvers and curers. Hospitals, particularly teaching hospitals, are where all the interesting problems are. As Professor Miller argues, 'there is an excessive concentration on the hospital as opposed to the community, and on the relatively small amount of serious illness that is treated in institutions, at the expense of attention to common causes of disablement'.

In fact, it is general practitioners who deal with between 90 and 95 per cent of all complaints taken to doctors. Furthermore, a 1973 study, *Present State and Future Needs of General Practice*, published by the Royal College of General Practitioners, showed that the illnesses GPs were consulted about were not the stuff of dramatic documentaries. They were, instead, predominantly minor ones, such as coughs, stomach upsets, tonsillitis and earache. These outnumbered tenfold complaints of major illnesses such as bronchitis and pneumonia. An average GP sees only one or two cases of cancer a year. A congenital abnormality could be expected only once in every five years.

Hospital doctors see themselves, and encourage others to see them, as an elite. Those in the teaching hospitals are, of course, a kind of super-elite, leaders of the medical world, shapers of medical education. These teachers become the role models for the future. To borrow Professor Miller's words, 'The company of biochemists and geneticists remains more stimulating and more attractive to the bright young medical man than that of social workers and chiropodists.' Indeed, since the creation of the NHS, the number of hospital doctors has increased by over 100 per cent, as has the number of nurses. Hospital specializations, techniques to advance self-worth and the appearance of need, now number 47, with 11 new ones having been created in the past ten years. This contrasts sharply with the state of affairs in primary and community care. The number of GPs has increased over the same period by only 36 per cent, and they account for only 6 per cent of the NHS budget. There are only about 1,000 community physicians to serve the whole of the United Kingdom while a large number of vacancies go unfilled. The school health service is woefully understaffed. There are a mere 46 doctors specializing in occupational health per 1 million workers.

Perhaps the final word on this point should rest with Professor

McKeown, whose book *The Role of Medicine* deserves the widest audience. He explains how the restricted nature of the work undertaken by teaching hospitals is a consequence of modern scientific medicine being grafted on to the secular voluntary hospitals of the eighteenth century. 'These hospitals limited their work to short-term remediable cases which were of greatest interest to the medical profession . . . Thus they excluded the majority of patients who had to be cared for in separate voluntary hospitals . . . or in public institutions (for the infectious, the mentally ill, and the destitute).' Scientific medicine, he argues, reinforced the element of selectivity, by encouraging the notion that the teaching of skills and techniques, to be practised on a small, carefully selected group of patients, was proper preparation for later medical practice.

The consequence is, Professor McKeown balefully notes, that, 'Professional interest is increasingly absorbed by methods of investigation and treatment whose complexities seem to challenge the attention of the best minds and whose rewards are assumed to justify it. The acute hospital is likely to become still more selective in its admission policies, and the teaching centre with its concentration of resources and abilities, will be the most exclusive of all. Doctors, nurses, and other health workers would then be trained in an environment which reveals a very limited part of the health task, an environment where prestige, rewards, and professional interest all seem to point in the same direction. After qualification, understandably, they will seek to continue in the activities which were the focus of their training, and only with the greatest reluctance will they consent to enter the massive neglected areas of health care. The large number of patients, particularly among the congenitally handicapped, the mentally ill and the aged sick . . . will be pushed further into the background, and the division of health services into two worlds will be even sharper than it is today.'

It should not come as a surprise that we have exported this same mentality to developing countries. The 1980 World Bank Report points to the emphasis these countries give to curative rather than preventive care, to the excessive construction of hospitals, and to the education of doctors which is often not geared to their countries' needs, but, rather, stresses rare diseases and the use of costly equipment while neglecting local health problems. Two-thirds of the health budget of most developing countries goes to medical education and teaching hospitals. In India, for example, I found doctors in the major teaching hospitals anxious to debate what care should be delivered to a severely handicapped new-born baby. And this in a country where 80 per cent of the population never see a doctor from birth till death, and where the infant mortality rate from poverty and infectious diseases is close to 1 in 5

The limitations of adopting this approach in developing countries are illustrated by a medical school programme in Colombia for the hospital care of premature infants. Survival rates were achieved which compared with those in the United States. But 70 per cent of the infants discharged were dead within three months because of infection, malnutrition and general poverty. United Medical Enterprises, which supplies hospitals and medical equipment to Middle East countries, reported 1979 sales at £20 million and pre-tax profits of £2 million. 'Business is brisk,' glowed the financial reporter of *The Times*. This company, 70 per cent of which is owned by the state-run National Enterprise Board, also operates in Jordan, Nigeria and the Ivory Coast and has recently ventured into Uganda. In each of these countries, the average life expectancy is about fifty years (as opposed to about seventy in the United Kingdom). Nigeria has an infant mortality rate of 163 per thousand (as compared with 16 per thousand in the United Kingdom), for which hospitals offer no solution, since the causes lie in poverty and the infectious diseases it brings in its wake. Uganda is still witnessing the starvation of its people in the north, which so shocked the world in 1980.

Let me now come to my seventh point. With the increasing emphasis on hospitals as the hub of medical care has come another unfortunate feature of modern medicine: that medicine is and should be an enterprise calling for the use of ever more advanced and complex technology. Christian Barnard filled the massive football stadium in Rio twice when he talked of how he performed the world's first heart transplant, yet the majority of his audience could not afford the simple medicine to rid themselves of their intestinal worms. And, in his own country, Oxfam was giving out measles vaccine to malnourished children whose lives were at risk from infection. Schweitzer, in his hospital in Lambarene, becomes a somewhat ludicrous figure, dissipating his energies, albeit for the most noble of reasons. Pressure on the French Government from someone of his stature could well have produced better results for the health of the people of equatorial Africa than losing himself in a primitive jungle hospital, trying to patch up broken lives.

More and more diagnostic aids, surgical tools and supportive equipment, ever more complex, not to mention drugs, the NHS bill for which in 1981 was over £1000 million, are pressed on doctors. The trend is as predictable as it is regrettable. If you are trained to think of yourself as an applied scientist and problem-solver, raised in an environment of white coats and machinery, where people are constantly being monitored and measured, it is inevitable that you will want the latest machine. Recourse to such technology is deemed entirely proper. And those who manufacture such machinery will ensure that the hospital realizes that, without this particular advanced scanner, or whatever, the care being offered may well be thought of as substandard. The combination of the administration's nervousness and the doctor's professional self-image is more than enough to ensure that the machine is categorized as essential, to be obtained as soon as possible.

In case you think the picture I am painting is a caricature, consider the NHS distinction awards, which are given to consultants as supplements to their salary. The three specialities most frequently rewarded are, thoracic surgeons, 73 per cent of whom receive awards, neurosurgeons, 67 per cent of whom get awards and cardiologists, 64 per cent of whom get awards. Consultants in geriatrics and mental health, two areas where the technological model fits poorly, although these two areas are blessed with by far the most patients, receive the fewest awards, only 23 and 25 per cent of them respectively. So government, with the aid of the profession, reinforces this technological approach to medicine which I am seeking to illustrate and criticize.

It is fair to say, however, that evidence is beginning to emerge that some at least are having second thoughts as to whether medicine ought to be riding this roller-coaster of advanced technology, not only because of the enormous financial costs involved but also in view of the cost in human terms. R.L. Himsworth, for instance, writing in 1975 in the book of essays *Specialized Futures*, was moved to remark that, 'At present the expensive enthusiasm for coronary care units is barely contained by administrative and financial considerations and not at all by the lack of evidence that they have a major effect on the overall mortality.' After all, what could be more stressful than to be in such a unit!

Professor Miller makes the same point: 'The wiring up of a patient with coronary thrombosis to his elaborate instrumentation is a pleasing exercise in technical virtuosity, but evidence of the superiority of the treatment of cardiac infarction in an intensive coronary unit over its simple management at home is not entirely convincing. In fact, the only clinical trial even hints that the opposite may be the case.'

Nowhere is the human cost of advanced technology more evident than when applied to those who are fatally ill and dying. Nowhere is the technological imperative of 'if we can do it, we must do it' more inappropriate. Heroic forms of intervention, in which the only hero is the patient, become the order of the day, despite doubts as to whether any benefit which may accrue outweighs the hardship endured. It should come as no surprise to learn that, of the vast amount of money spent on health care in the United States, close to 3 billion dollars, 60 per cent is spent on care in the last year of life.

And a further objection is, of course, that technology represents a short-term solution to what are long-term problems. Indeed, to concentrate attention and resources on a form of medicine which reacts to illness already caused means that less interest is cultivated in seeking to discover the origin and causes of a particular illness, and less effort is available to do so. Such a choice between these two approaches to medical care arose, in effect, in the case of polio. At one stage, a decision had to be made whether further research effort and resources should be concentrated on the development of better iron lungs, on the hypothesis that polio was an inevitable incidence of life, or whether they should be spent on the search for a polio vaccine. Those advocating the second alternative finally, and not without difficulty, won the day, with the result that polio is no longer the scourge it was.

The fact remains, however, that the lure of advanced technology is irresistible to the doctor, serving as both validation and vindication of his training and of his image of himself as really the applied scientist, problem-solver and curer. It is this same mentality which fuels the search for so-called wonder drugs. Though doctors may well frown at the term, the pursuit goes on regardless. Medical research exerts a spell over governments and foundations and thus over the public. The spell is that something is just around the corner, a breakthrough is imminent. We are all mesmerized and the premise largely goes unquestioned, namely that scientific medicine, with its accompanying technology, is the proper way.

Even respected writers can fall into the trap. Take, for instance, the headline 'Is breast cancer next for treatment breakthrough?' which accompanied an article by Dr Tony Smith, the former medical correspondent of *The Times*, on 21 February 1980, in which he described what he called 'the battle against breast cancer'. Interferon, an agent produced by the body and alleged to have therapeutic properties, is the latest candidate. It would of course be wonderful if it were true, but the record of wonder drugs has not been good since the 1950s.

Something by way of an aside is to inquire why interferon warrants scholarly attention while laetrile, the subject of so much controversy in the United States, is condemned. Laetrile is a vitaminic substance, vitamin B17, derived principally from apricot stones. A large number of States, including California, have laws making its sale unlawful. Some, however, claim it as a valuable aid in the treatment of cancer. The medical establishment and the Federal Government's Food and Drug Administration take another view — that its therapeutic value is unproven, that its ingredients make it potentially dangerous and that a patient may delay or even forgo recourse to other accepted forms of cancer therapy and thus not receive the benefit these could bring. To them it is just a modern form of snake oil.

The difference in response cannot be for lack of proof about laetrile: neither it nor interferon has been tested by traditional methods. Nor can it be merely the toxicity of laetrile. It is no more toxic than other substances commonly used in the chemotherapy of patients with cancer. Can it be that laetrile is associated with the counter-culture parodied as vegetarian, sandal-wearing socialists? Can it be that the medical establishment and drug companies are apprehensive about the call for a patient's freedom to act as he wishes as regards his own illness? After all, an estimated $20,000 million a year are spent in the United States on conventional cancer therapy — surgery, irradiation and drugs. Can it be that doctors see the advocacy of laetrile as a threat to their exclusive power, not only to treat disease but also to control the forms of treatment to be used?

My eighth, and final, point concerning the inappropriateness of the way medicine is perceived concerns the notion of illness. I have already spent some time considering this notion and here will confine myself to two matters.

The first is the extent to which the notion of illness has been expanded. We have seen that at base illness is a socially determined and evaluative term susceptible of being put to different uses, so as to confer or deny the status of 'ill' on suitable candidates. The growing categorization of perceptions and circumstances as illnesses has been a feature of the past decades. Much of this expansion has come through the notion of labelling, through the application of taxonomical skills. It does not follow, of course, that because X can now be divided into Y and Z this necessarily represents any advance in knowledge as to how these come about and what can be done about them.

Nowhere is this more true than in the area of mental illness. Indeed, an argument can be made for the proposition that the categories of mental illness came first, the product of theorizing, and only later did there emerge a growing army of people to fill these categories. But the process is not limited to mental illness. The response to many of the problems of old age — which are, in fact, problems of, for example, relative poverty, lack of adequate heating, and social isolation — has been to treat them as separate, quite unrelated illnesses, and thereby to medicalize them. The elderly are seen as ill. The consequence is that resources are directed to the provision of doctors, nurses and hospital beds, rather than to redressing the social ills the elderly encounter. In the process, not only is it probable that more money is ultimately spent than would otherwise be necessary, but also the elderly are denied the opportunity to retain the dignity that illness so easily robs them of.

Another example is the ambivalence shown by medicine towards pregnancy, whether to regard it as a normal state or as having at least some of the attributes of illness. Alan Davis, in his book *Relationships between Doctors and Patients,* cautions against the 'evangelical approach' to antenatal care. Doctors, he suggests, feel obliged to justify their tests on the grounds of possible risks and dangers, and then have to spend inordinate lengths of time reassuring pregnant women and persuading them that all is well and that pregnancy is quite natural.

A final example is the resort to mass-screening devices to discover those 'at risk', who will, of course, be suitably apprehensive in the future, particularly if little or nothing can be done once the knowledge is gained. The report in the *Daily Telegraph* of 15 September 1979 of Dr d'Souza's work at St Thomas's Hospital Medical School in London has not dampened the enthusiasm for such tests, particularly on the part of those who would profit by them. Dr d'Souza's seven-year study concluded that regular medical examinations to detect disease at an early stage were an expensive and inefficient way of raising standards of health. Not surprisingly, the Director of Research for BUPA, the leading commercial scheme for the provision of private medical care in the United Kingdom, was quick to criticize the nature of the research and its results. Only three months earlier, BUPA reported that a survey it had conducted had shown that, on average, 540 electricians were less healthy than business managers who were twelve years older. Although this finding could encourage resort to doctors, it is not immediately clear what the doctors would be able to do about it.

One startling use of screening is that now being used in a number of western countries, and, particularly, in the United States by certain chemical companies, as reported in the *New York Times* of 3 February 1980. Workers seeking employment are screened for their suscepti-bility to various chemical agents. Those categorized as 'hyper-susceptibles' are 'weeded out', even though they are within the normal range of human variations. Critics see this as an improper attempt to divert attention from the dangerous conditions of the workplace by blaming the ills that the worker is exposed to on his genes. They point to Aldous Huxley's prophecy of this in *Brave New World,* in which workers were 'trained' to tolerate toxic chemicals.

The expansion of the notion of illness also meets a social need. It allows us to sweep under the social rug whole groups of people who are otherwise a nuisance. They may not seek to be categorized as ill. Indeed they may resist or resent it. But, if doctors are prepared to say that particular forms of behaviour, or merely the incidents of growing old, are indeed illnesses, who are we to protest? The twinge of guilt we may feel about neglecting our fellow men, or even locking them away, is salved by the reassuring knowledge that they are ill and are now in the best possible hands in the circumstances. And, provided we keep our hospitals for the mentally ill and long-stay patients out in the backwoods, and their hostels in the decaying urban centres — indeed, anywhere but in our own particular neighbourhood — we can keep up this fiction. In fact, we have in this way created a separate society for the dispossessed and disadvantaged. Forgotten or underprivileged patients are looked after in these institutions by doctors and nurses from overseas, while the menial work is also done by immigrants — 'The underprivileged caring for each other in mutual under-standing', as Michael Wilson puts it in his book *Health is for People.* Or is it mutual resentment? You may be intrigued to learn, by the way, that the domestic running costs, just food, laundry, cleaning and so on, of an average mental hospital are about one-third of those of a London teaching hospital. That many are there in the first place is bad enough; that they should be so shabbily dealt with demonstrates the extent of the neglect.

Let me now turn to my second point concerning the notion of illness. It has, with disease, become the central concern of modern medicine. If we were to start all over again to design a model for modern medicine, most of us, I am sure, would opt for a design which concerned itself far, far more with the pursuit and preservation of health, of well-being. What we have instead is the very opposite: a system of medicine which reacts, which responds, which waits to pick up the broken pieces – a form of medicine, in short, concerned with illness, not health. A moment's thought demonstrates the folly of this. But the interests which combine to produce this state of affairs are too well entrenched for any redirection to be accomplished easily. Nonetheless, the significance of the present state of medicine should not be underestimated. It conditions the way we spend huge sums of money each year, roughly 6 per cent of our gross domestic product. It conditions the way we think of ourselves. It goes to the root of our value system, our cultural and social heritage. Meanwhile, debates go on among the medical profession as to how many doctors we should be producing. Concern is expressed at the threat posed to existing doctors' livelihoods by a possible glut of doctors. No one stops to say that these questions cannot be answered until the far more fundamental question is tackled: what should modern medicine be doing? The Report of the Royal Commission on the NHS contents itself with the rather Delphic utterance that 'the planned output of medical graduates is about right'. No clue is offered as to how this conclusion is arrived at. No indication is given that the Royal Commission even understood that what was involved in such a calculation was a set of profound social and political considerations.

Equally, in the United States, the *New York Times* reported on 2 September 1980 that the 'Government takes steps to Avert Glut of Doctors'. The Graduate Medical Education National Advisory Committee after four years of study has predicted that there will be 59,000 more doctors than needed by 1990 and 130,000 too many by the year 2000. The calculations are based, of course, on the assumption that medicine will continue to take its present form and that use of doctors by the population will be on the same basis as at present. Again, there seems to be no realization that such calculations are worthless without first considering the question of what role medicine should have. Furthermore, the Committee is able to warn of this glut while at the same time noticing that in certain regions of the country, and in certain types of medical care, especially lower-paying family practice and other primary care, severe shortages of doctors exist. This maldistribution of doctors, this co-existence of plenty with need, must make assertions of an oversupply ring hollow to many. The way in which modern medicine has developed is, in large part, responsible for this. How it is to be solved is a problem for the future. If it is to be solved, it may be that the claim that there are too many doctors will need to be reconsidered. It may be more accurate to say that there are too many doctors doing the wrong things.

These are some of the ways in which medicine has taken the wrong path. They are, of course, painted with the broad brush. It is important to realize that I am not denying that every day up and down the country wonderful things are being done. Despite this, could the nation's health be better, or if not better then no worse, at some gain, financial and social, to the citizenry if medicine took a different form? But the present state of medicine will take some changing. It is cultivated by the medical profession. It flatters the self-esteem of the doctor to see himself as the applied scientist and problem-solver spreading health. The present state of medicine has readily been adopted by a lay public, persuaded naively that herein lies the path to health, and with expectations which may be unwarranted but which are, of course, a product of the claims made by medicine. But, although this state of affairs may seem to satisfy the aspirations of the doctor to see himself as the applied scientist and problem-solver satisfied.

For a start, the cost of financing medicine in the form it now takes is clearly beyond what we are willing to pay in the form of taxation. We complain if we are asked to forgo anything, but we vote for promises of reduced taxation and reduced public spending. Of course, the dissatisfaction doctors feel, as rising national costs are reflected in their income tax, is tinged with a professional reluctance to countenance any cuts in expenditure on medical care. Indeed, as a group they are voluble, for example, in their demand for the so-called freedom to prescribe, whatever the cost. If drugs were prescribed under their general chemical name rather than under a specific company's brand name, the NHS would make a considerable saving, estimated to be at least £25 million a year by R. Barry O'Brien, in his important series of articles in the *Daily Telegraph* of November 1979. Yet doctors resist such an obvious financial control as an unconscionable interference in their rights. No one seems to stop to ask where such rights come from, if not from us.

It should be said that the GP's position is not an easy one. The Royal Commission reports that they are 'subjected to massive pressure from the drug companies. A study in 1974-5 showed that a typical GP may be exposed to over 1,300 advertisements for 250 drugs each month. In 1977 the cost of sales promotion in the United Kingdom by drug companies was about £71 million, most of it aimed at GPs. The relative isolation of many GPs from pharmacologist and clinical colleagues adds to their problems in evaluating this mountain of material.' As O'Brien points out, this promotion amounted by 1979 to a staggering £1,458 for each doctor in Britain. Furthermore, the practice is growing of GPs being offered discounts and bonuses by drug companies to promote certain drugs, as *The Times* of 12 April 1980 notes in its report of a speech by John Kerr, the former President of the Pharmaceutical Society of Great Britain. These practices, he warned, were being reflected in the prescribing habits of some GPs. This is a commonplace in the United States. For instance, in 1974 the Senate Labour and Welfare Committee, chaired by Senator Edward Kennedy, reported that in 1974 drug companies spent an average of between $3,000 and $5,000 on each physician in the United States. This money was spent merely on sales promotion through gifts of such items as pocket calculators, pens, freezers, and televisions. Some of these were outright gifts, some were bonuses to reward doctors for prescribing a particular drug. In addition, the Committee reported that 2,000 million free drug samples were sent to doctors. Indeed, it is not unusual for a drug company in the United States to spend 15 – 20 per cent of its annual sales revenue on promotion and advertising, a proportion considerably larger than non-drug companies. In the United Kingdom also, 15 per cent of sales revenue on average is devoted to promotion while between 7 and 12 per cent is spent on research and development.

Ever more expensive equipment is a further cause of spiralling costs. Yet, doctors are among the first to urge that it be acquired. Also, albeit with less stridency, they can be heard arguing the need for better conditions for hospital patients. And finally, of course, when it comes to their pay, they have not been slow to keep themselves at or near the head of the professional league, while at the same time insisting on the right to private practice in addition. The bitter comment attributed to Aneurin Bevan, the Minister of Health in the post-war Government, that to win over the consultants to the cause of the NHS he had 'choked their mouths with gold', echoes down the years.

A second reason for dissatisfaction with the state of modern medicine is that we, the public, have been led to expect too much and have been more than willing partners in the process. We have come almost to believe in magic cures and the waving of wands. The reality is a constant disappointment. The promised or expected cures are not there. We are also disappointed for another reason. The simple fact is that for large numbers of people the many and varied services offered by medicine are just not available. And I do not mean here the interventionist, hospital-based medicine I have criticized. I mean the preventive and primary care which large segments of the population do not have ready access to and which, if it were accompanied by other appropriate social and political measures, would help them pursue and enjoy more healthy lives. I will return to this theme at much greater length later. Now, I will merely refer you to the Report of the Royal Commission on the NHS which makes the general point most clearly:

'In some declining urban areas and in parts of London in particular the National Health Service is failing dismally to provide an adequate primary care system to its patients.' Dr Brian Jarman's *Report on Health Care in Inner London*, issued in the spring of 1981 confirms this in depressing detail. 'Since the establishment of the NHS,' the Royal Commission Report goes on, 'the position of those in social classes 4 and 5 appears to have worsened relative to those in social classes 1 and 2.'

Now more than ever, wealthier means healthier. Indeed, it is hard to criticize those who argue that the structure of medical education and health care is organized so as to legitimate a form of society in which concern for the weak may be expressed, but is translated into action in a fashion which is limited at best. Illness, then, they argue, on this analysis, is not perceived as being a consequence of poverty, wretched living conditions and unfulfilled lives. Illness is separate from and causes these. The tables are turned on the poor. As Frederick Gates, the first Director of the Rockefeller Foundation, wrote, 'misery is a technical not a social problem'. Medicine can thus be conceived of as an apolitical, value-free enterprise, a technical enterprise unrelated to the political circumstances of the society in which it is practised. Inequalities or injustices become problems for others, if problems at all, while medicine goes on its blinkered way.

A final reason for dissatisfaction is the role the doctor finds himself playing. Reality casts him in a far different role from the one which he has been trained to expect and perform. A tension is produced between the model and the reality. It has severe repercussions on the morale of many doctors. Take the general practitioner. A large part of his daily clientele are people who quite simply are unhappy. In the absence of anyone else to go to, and in view of the ready availability of the general practitioner and the extended notion of illness cultivated by doctors, the unhappy person diagnoses himself as ill and then goes to his GP. But many GPs feel they are trained to treat those who are 'really ill'. This is what those years of white coats and science have prepared them for. They think their time is being wasted and, more significantly, they feel impotent in the face of the unhappiness being complained of. A 1977 survey, by Cartwright and Anderson, referred to in the Royal Commission's Report, showed that a third of all recently qualified GPs felt that they should not have to deal with their patients' family problems and that it was not appropriate for people to seek such help from their GPs.

To do something, the doctor, with varying degrees of reluctance, confers on them the accolade of illness. He then commonly prescribes tranquillizers. With the other regularly used mood-changing drugs, these account for about 10 per cent of all prescriptions. Indeed, even the makers of Valium, Hoffman-La-Roche, hardly famous for public-spiritedness, were constrained in August 1980 to advise doctors in the United States not to prescribe it for the ordinary stresses of life (whatever that may mean), and similar Department of Health guide-lines were published in March 1980 in the *British Medical Journal*. As I have already indicated, the GP thus finds himself playing the part of socializing agent, ensuring that, whatever form the unhappiness or dissatisfaction take, they are kept in check, and whatever pain there is, it is not felt, even if this means that the social and economic conditions which give rise to them remain unaddressed. Alternatively, the GP finds himself faced by those beset by today's common ills. He is in danger of becoming the victim of his own hyperbole, in that he is asked to work wonders when there are none to work. The damage has been done. There are only symptoms to ease, parts to patch. The frustration is inevitable.

Then consider the doctors who work in hospital. If traumatic injury and perhaps some aspects of obstetrics are put aside, hospitals are now largely engaged in two tasks, neither of which remotely conforms to the image of modern medicine represented by the teaching hospital. One task is that of serving as dumping-grounds for the old and so-called mentally ill. The hospital is little more than a hotel or hostel. The frustration of the doctor, trained to see himself not as a carer but as a solver, is obvious and it can only increase as the elderly come to form an even greater proportion of the population. Indeed, quite whether doctors, as trained at present, have a role to play at all in such hospitals, or whether others could not do the job just as well, is a question which presses for an answer.

The other task doctors in hospitals are performing is that of calling upon more and more complex and expensive technology to respond to situations in which, when one looks at the general overall picture, there is usually little that can be done. To use the metaphor of the mechanic, the tyre can be patched, but even so it is permanently weak. I know well that there are some who will say, 'It is all very well talking in general terms, but I have got Mr A who is clamouring for help, or Miss B whom I may be able to help. Then there is old Mrs C's hip operation, and Mr D's hernia to fix. I cannot tell them to think of the generality of care, I have a duty to them.'

I concede much of this. But let me make two points. First, I am not advocating that we burn down our hospitals tomorrow. Of course, we need our marvellous accident units, our general medicine and surgery, whether it be for hips or hernias, haemorrhoids or Hodgkin's disease. But, even here, I wonder how much more rewarding and beneficial it would be to work towards preventing, for example, the degeneration of the hip, or to concentrate on other preventive measures, such as a production system which does not give productivity bonuses, nor uses piece-rates, in industries in which these are known to be associated with an increase in work accidents. How much more rewarding these measures would be than to have units waiting to pick up the pieces and work wonders in sewing the parts together so that the seams are barely visible. If such preventive strategies as these were pursued, greater attention could be paid to the marvellous developments, for example, in aiding those with ailing sight or hearing, where the benefits conferred are more than short-term or palliative and where the numbers who could be helped are so great.

My second point is that, put baldly, certain services simply should not be offered until matters of greater priority are dealt with. We have to meet head on the sort of argument advanced in a recent letter to *The Times* from a doctor. 'A dying man', Dr Jessop wrote, 'does not care that facilities can only benefit a tiny fraction of those patients whose lives might be salvaged. The chance of being among them is all he's got.' There are perfectly respectable ethical theories which, in the context of harsh choices, such as those we face now (and always will as regards resources), allow for conduct which will benefit the larger or more worthy number, even if this inevitably means others may suffer. One example was the decision taken by the Surgeon-General of the United States in the Second World War in North Africa, that only those who, on recovery, would be able to fight again should receive scarce penicillin. Thus, those 'wounded' in brothels received penicillin; those wounded badly in military engagements did not. Another was the decision taken in Uganda in 1980 to feed only those starving children who may recover, leaving the rest to die.

Our situation is not so desperate, but the same principle must apply. Indeed, such decisions are made every day in the NHS when resources come to be allocated. As Michael Wilson, a doctor and theologian, argued recently, in *Health is for People*, 'only when we are prepared to let some people die will we be free to make more humane decisions in the distribution of resources. Our fear of death leads us to use death as the final incontrovertible argument.' We are prepared to ignore much human misery for the prospect of saving a few lives. John James, Assistant Secretary at the Department of Health and Social Security in charge of planning, remarked recently that consultants, opposed to shifts of resources from the well-endowed areas to the Cinderella areas of geriatrics and mental illness, have not been averse to using 'shroud-waving tactics'.

Well, after these rather harsh words about the wrong emphasis adopted by modern medicine, the wrong path it has taken, I shall consider in the next chapter how the emphasis should be shifted — what a better path for the future may be.

3 Suffer the little children

It is hard to avoid the conclusion that the NHS has failed us. This is a grave charge, given the money, energy, time and dedication expended. But, I repeat, the NHS has failed us. I say this for two reasons. First, the NHS has so organized medicine that it is barely recognizable as a health service. It has to that extent failed us. Certainly it has failed to take its opportunities. When we consider the pursuit of health beyond that which medicine can affect, here too the NHS has not been mobilized to achieve this end. It has not become the focus of action in Government planning and policies aimed at improving health. Successive Governments have thereby failed us. It must be our task to make it clear to Government and those who manage and control medicine, that we are not content to watch our health care services merely tick over at their present level, far less to watch them slowly disintegrate. There can and must be improvements and it is our responsibility to ensure that they happen.

I have already drawn the distinction between the extent to which medicine can affect health by responding to illness through cures (rarely), palliation or prevention, and those aspects of health which are the product of social and political forces. Both of these aspects of health could be regarded as within the proper purview of the NHS and the Department of Health. But in both regards, I look at what has been done and find it wanting, whether it is the type of medical care provided or the type of society we build and the commitment we make to health. The two aspects are, of course, inevitably interwoven. Attitudes towards what medicine involves and can do clearly influence decisions about what other measures are appropriate, or whose responsibility they may be. To separate the two is not always easy but it may assist in better analysing what has happened and what could be done. It will also allow us to see and understand clearly the limits and limitations of medicine. What a boon this last point would be for doctors, who so often feel impotent before requests to work miracles. What a boon it would be, if only they could overcome the professional suspicion that causes them to see threats behind any analysis.

What I propose to put before you is a blueprint for change and improvement. It is in two parts. I shall suggest some strategies which would improve health, first through medical care and then other means. They will, however, be difficult in the extreme to achieve. Though obvious to the committed, they challenge received wisdom and the established order of things. They necessarily involve deep and thorough-going political changes. They are addressed to the structure of society rather than merely to modifications within that structure. Let me say at the outset that mine is a view of measured pessimism. I do not expect to see improvements, of the sort we all realize are required, implemented in the immediate future. But it is still important constantly to present the arguments and hope thereby to sow some seeds of change.

Let me now turn to the blueprint. The first part is directed towards the reorientation and redirection of medical care. It calls for action by doctors, by those who manage medicine and by Government. It can be broken down into a series of points. The first is that medicine must take a new path. We have seen already some of the ways in which it has taken the wrong path. With the decline of serious threats to health from infections, our health-care system has turned away from environmental considerations towards the notion of personal health care. It has become an illness service rather than a health service. This is not to say that modern health care can do nothing for us; it can, and does, provide many much-needed services. But it could do far, far more if a different balance were struck, a balance which would make it more properly a health service.

All too often, it has become a system of symptom swatting. To alter this, to shift the emphasis of medical care towards primary preventive care and the promotion of health, is the task and the challenge facing those who control medicine and those who practise it. While I remain a convinced and committed supporter of the NHS and view proposed alternatives to it with distaste and no little trepidation, I feel it has become harnessed to the wrong tasks. And we, of course, have let this happen. I, and many others, have argued this for years, not without criticism, for powerful forces stand in the way, whether the vested interests of some sections of the medical profession, the skewed image of medicine we have all acquired, or the lobbying of those whose commercial interests lie in medicine retaining its present nature (only always more so). Besides these forces, it could be thought that a further obstacle to change stands in the way. The present political climate seems hardly auspicious. A time of major economic difficulties would seem an inappropriate one in which to recommend improvements in the health services, if only because it is assumed that such improvements would cost money. This is, of course, not necessarily so. In the short term, cost may be the same (or at worst slightly increased) but it will be distributed in a different manner. In the long term money may even be saved.

For instance, money spent in reducing the number of accidents at work or on the road is money gained in terms of reduced hospital and health-care use, in reduced social security payments and increased economic productivity. What is more, this preoccupation with costs suggests that money is the only value. That it is important is clear; that it is the only value is nonsense.

My second point follows from this. We must curb our predilection for medicine in the form of ever more complex technology. Note, I do not say abandon it. But we must keep it and its advocates, doctors and commercial entrepreneurs, under our control. Hospitals with their massive costs, expensive equipment and commitment to technology have elbowed themselves into the centre of the medical stage, consuming now some 65 per cent of available health-care resources. The debate in the United Kingdom during the autumn of 1980, and again in the summer of 1982, concerning the merits of heart transplants offers a useful lesson. It was conducted largely by doctors, as if what was at stake was a narrow technical matter, instead of a profound question as to the proper direction of our health-care resources. In reality, heart transplants are only an example, and, because of their rarity and relative uselessness, virtually an irrelevance. There are after all 400 deaths a day in the United Kingdom from heart disease. The real debate is much wider. It concerns advanced technology, interventionist, last-ditch, patch-and-repair medicine, as against other measures aimed at reducing the need for such intervention. The debate should not be in terms of 'either . . . or'. It must be in terms of 'How much of each do we need and can we afford?'

Quite clearly, we need, and have come to rely on, medical technology in the treatment of kidney disease, in aiding the blind and deaf, in avoiding the birth of deformed and disabled babies and in many other areas. What we do not need, and must guard against, is a mentality which conceives of medical care only, or primarily, in terms of such technological approaches. Instead, we need to direct more of our energy and resources towards the promotion of good health. One tragic but often overlooked feature of the defence of heart transplant surgery is that it is so clearly an example of the crazy contradictions of our society. We can only transplant hearts if we have otherwise healthy corpses from which to take them. Where do we get such corpses? We depend on the appalling death rate from road accidents, most of which are eminently preventable.

The next point in this part of the blueprint is one that cannot be emphasized too much. We have already seen that change and improvement need not cost more. It is important now that we notice the obverse of this. The mere provision of more and more money will not of itself improve the quality of our health care. Unfavourable comparisons have been made between the proportion of gross domestic product spent in the United Kingdom on health care, and that spent by the United States or West Germany. In 1977, the proportion was 5.6 per cent in the United Kingdom as against 6.7 per cent in Germany and 7.4 per cent in the United States. By 1979, the United States proportion had grown with startling rapidity to over 9 per cent, and by 1981 to 9.8, an increase of 15 per cent just in 1980. In England and Germany, it was about 6 and 7 per cent respectively by 1979. Both Germany and the United States also had proportionately more doctors than the United Kingdom. But the Royal Commission on the NHS cautions against using such comparisons as the basis for any 'sweeping assertions'. For example, the latest available figures show that both West Germany and the United States, despite their greater expenditure on health care, have a worse record in terms of perinatal and maternal mortality than England and Wales and no better record in life expectancy.

It is trite to remark that it is not the amount of money but how it is spent which is significant. If, for example, we continue to think of health care in terms which give pride of place, as regards resources, to hospitals, we could easily find ourselves spending more and more, with no great benefit to the overall health of the nation. Furthermore, as Dr Draper's Unit for the Study of Health Policy, at Guy's Hospital, London, argues in its 1978 pamphlet, *The NHS in the next 30 years*, short-term increases in financial outlay may well be offset by longer-term financial gain produced by reduced use of health care resources by a healthier population, increased productivity and prosperity, and reduced rates of crime and vandalism.

I turn now to my fourth point. One of the declared aims of the major reorganization of the NHS in 1974 was the integration of individual with community care. The result has been less than successful. The second reorganization (or upheaval) of 1982 holds out no prospect of improvement. Primary care is on the verge of collapse in some areas. Where it functions, it may not be meeting the real needs of the community. If GPs were more adequately prepared for the real health needs of their patients, which are as much to do with social problems as with particular diseases, then the beginnings of a movement towards better health could emerge. Progress is undoubtedly being made now that post-graduate training for those intending to be GPs became compulsory in 1981. Indeed the GP could well become an important focus for the sort of social reform necessary to produce the improvement in health we claim we desire. He is the central pivot of the health care service. He well recognizes much of what I am arguing, but for too long his voice has not been heard over the clamour of the hospital doctor or the medical politician. No one is better placed to gauge the social pressures and problems of the day and pass the news on up the line, and no one is better placed to act as an educator for better health and pass the word down the line.

Besides the primary care of the GP, there is the need for greater emphasis on community medicine. The reorganization of the NHS introduced on All Fools' Day 1974, as H.A.Waldron notes in his book *The Medical Role in Environmental Health*, destroyed the long tradition of the much-valued medical officer of health, whose major concern was public health, and launched the newly created community physicians on uncharted seas. They were soon sucked into administration and became largely concerned with personal care rather than public health. The net result has been unfilled posts, disenchantment, and reluctance of newly qualified doctors to go anywhere near the job. The decline of community medicine in training and as a career has meant that half the present community physicians were qualified before 1950 and three-quarters before 1955. And in a study published in 1976, in the *British Medical Journal*, by J. Parkhouse and C. McLaughlin, out of 2,022 newly qualified doctors, only 10 put community medicine as their first choice for a career. It can be hoped that the 1982 reorganization of the NHS, by giving the District Medical Officer greater status and independence, will go some way to reversing this unfortunate trend. Whether it will bring about any revitalization in this branch of medicine remains to be seen.

No one, after all, can really doubt that a substantial contribution to health could be made by someone whose job it is, as community physicians in Oxford put it in their evidence to the Royal Commission on the NHS, to be responsible for 'highlighting the health problems in his particular population, for stimulating different health professionals to plan their services to meet these problems, and for evaluating and monitoring the success of these services'. One example may make the point. Claims that hospital use has been reduced and money thereby saved by the earlier discharge of patients, particularly the elderly and mentally ill, ring hollow if on examination it is clear that the services in the community, which are then supposed to take over, are just not adequate to the task, so that the patient must be re-admitted or languish alone and neglected.

This same understaffing and general demoralization is reflected in other areas of community health. The school health services are woefully ill equipped to engage in the kind of thorough preventive care and health education which would pay such dividends in the child's later life. The Report of the Court Committee on Child Health Services in 1976 drew particular attention to the 'failure of the school health service to give adequate attention to health education'. Occupational health is another example of a missed opportunity. Its aim is to promote health at work and thereby reduce accidents and injuries. It is a subject which is neglected in medical training. As Waldron points out, there are only 46 specialist industrial doctors per million male workers. Under the departmental umbrella of the Department of Employment and separated from the NHS, occupational health and safety stumble along while accidents at work kill 650 people a year and an estimated million are injured and require time off. To take just one example, 1 in 5 cotton-spinning workers suffers from byssinosis, a crippling, progressive and incurable disease caused by toxic dust. Some 6000 workers are thought to have the disease and one worker a week who dies had it. 'Steadfastly ignored by factory inspectors, employers and trade unions,' *The Times* of 17 August 1982 reports, 'it has none the less been running in epidemic proportions in Lancashire mill-towns for more than a century,' although well known, I would add, to specialists in occupational health for as long.

It follows, then, and this is my next point, that, important as the emphasis on primary and community care may be, even greater emphasis must be placed by our health service in the future on two interrelated exercises — the prevention of illness and accidents and the promotion of health. Since I lay great stress on this, let us be clear from the beginning what I am saying. I do not see preventive care as some panacea for all our ills. Furthermore, I readily concede, as I have already said, that we need, and must not neglect, many of our existing medical services. I do not advocate that we become therapeutic nihilists, and decry everything that goes by the name of medicine today. Indeed, as Muir Gray points out in his excellent book *Man Against Disease*, some take the view that prevention has three phases. First, you can prevent disease — primary prevention; then you can prevent the effects of disease, by treatment at an early stage — secondary prevention; and third, you can prevent the serious consequences of disease by further treatment — tertiary prevention. Curative medicine may be concerned with prevention at the secondary and tertiary stages. So it is not a question of either curative medicine or preventive medicine, as some would make it seem. It is rather a question of where along the spectrum you concentrate most resources.

In my view, for us to have a sane health care policy, we must concentrate much more on primary preventive medicine. If this means, as it inevitably must, that some aspects of modern curative care must be neglected or abandoned, then so be it. The benefits to be gained outweigh any loss. It will mean that profound changes will have to be made. The mentality adopted towards medical care, illness and health by doctors and laymen alike must change, research must redirect itself, at least in part, and resources must be reallocated on a considerable scale. That the chapter in the Royal Commission's Report on the NHS which dealt with these issues was the shortest, bar one, in the whole Report suggests that the process of change may not be easy.

The first essential step in any process towards redirecting effort or reallocating resources is to see how these are at present distributed. It is no rhetorical device to describe the disparities in the present provision of health care among the various groups in our society as a scandal. The provision of health care rests on political and social decisions. The political values which are supposed to be at the heart of any decisions made for the provision of health care are well known — that need should be the sole criterion of receipt of service and that funds should be raised on the basis of ability to contribute. Though these values have not been formally rejected as principles, commitment to them has certainly wavered. Indeed, the provision of health care in practice has seen a systematic and widespread departure from them. The evidence has been available for a long time. *Inequalities in Health*, the 1980 report compiled by a group under the chairmanship of Sir Douglas Black, President of the Royal College of Physicians, is the latest and most impressive account to appear. In the dry language of such reports, the group found 'marked inequalities in health between the social classes in Britain'.

J. Tudor Hart wrote in the *Lancet* of 27 February 1971, of an 'inverse care law' which provides that where there is most sickness and death, GPs have the largest number of patients, the heaviest work load and the least hospital support. Simply put, not only must there be a major shift of emphasis towards preventive care, but this care also must reach those who need it most, the poor and the disadvantaged. I shall return shortly to the situation in which the poor find themselves, since it illustrates perfectly the overlap between the first part of this blueprint, the contribution medicine can make, and the second, the need for structural change aimed at improving health. For it must be obvious that the poor are caught in a spiral of deprivation, with one hardship lending momentum to, or bringing about, the next. It must be obvious, for example, that developing preventive care in, say, antenatal care, is useless if the woman cannot find the time, or money, for travel to avail herself of the service.

Any call for a shift of emphasis towards preventive care does not go unopposed. In one sense, preventive care is like motherhood. Who could be against it? So its opponents, or those who would keep it in its rightful place (at the back of the queue), take a more subtle approach. One argument put forward by those anxious to maintain the existing emphasis on interventionist medicine is that you cannot prevent illness, or promote health, until you know what causes illness or ill health. And, to discover causes, you need the sort of medicine practised now, backed by technology and research. There is, of course, some truth in this. The argument goes on that we simply do not yet know what causes the common illnesses which afflict and kill us, with perhaps the exceptions of smoking and its relationship with lung cancer, and alcohol with liver damage. The implication is that, until we do, medicine should continue in its present form. Consider, for example, the fact that, in the United States, mortality from heart disease has declined in recent years, concurrently with an increase in exercise and a great reduction in smoking. Yet arguments about the

54

role played by eating fat, or exercising, or smoking, in heart disease still continue.

The *Times Health Supplement* of 26 February 1982 refers to research published in the United States in the *Journal of the American Medical Association* showing an age-adjusted drop of about a quarter in heart diseases in the decade ending in 1979. The research supports the belief that a combination of changes in diet, smoking, treatment of high blood pressure and increased exercise have contributed to the decline. 'In contrast', the report goes on, 'in England and Wales, where there has been much scepticism and "scientific" doubt and apathy about preventive efforts involving diet and vigorous control of hypertension, mortality figures have remained depressingly constant. Among middle-aged men in 1968, the chances of a coronary heart disease death in an American was 40 per cent higher than that of an Englishman, while by 1976 the American risk had actually declined to below that of the English.'

Indeed, if we are to wait until the perfect controlled experiment has demonstrated that it is factor X which is the real killer, preventive medicine will have to await the millennium. Besides, it must be obvious by now that research aimed at isolating individual causative agents is of doubtful validity, since there are few modern afflictions which can be traced to one particular cause. There are after all good historical precedents for taking action to prevent illness without the ability to justify the action scientifically. When in 1853 John Snow removed the handle of the Broad Street water pump in Soho, he could not prove the link between the water and cholera. Indeed, the prevailing theory was that cholera was carried by foul air. But, once the pump handle was removed, the cholera did not spread. Equally, we can now observe that people who are obese seem more prone to illness, and most of us know what makes us fat. Indeed, insurance underwriters, those most hard-headed of people, follow a simple rule. The more overweight you are, the higher the premium they demand. They do not wait until the scientific finger can be pointed at this or that specific causative factor. So, while I concede the value of some modern interventionist medicine, in terms of the information and insights it may offer, this does not persuade me that it must be supported in all its various forms, or that preventive care must necessarily play second fiddle to it.

It is fair to say, however, that even if medical care took the path I have suggested, improvements in the general health of the nation would not be so very great, although they would undoubtedly be significant. This is because, as I have argued, the power of medicine and those who practise it to influence health is, in large part, limited by the realities of the world beyond medicine, which they cannot control and only barely influence. Aaron Wildavsky, the American political scientist, captures the point perfectly in what could serve as the creed, or basic premise, of this part of the blueprint: 'According to the Great Equation, medical care equals health. But the Great Equation is wrong . . . The best estimates are that the medical system affects about 10 per cent of the usual indices for measuring health . . . the remaining 90 per cent are determined by factors over which doctors have little or no control, from individual life style . . . to social conditions . . . to the physical environment.'

This is no criticism of doctors. No one expects them to be able to reshape society so as to improve health. It is important, however, that the doctor does not react by proposing that we revert to the exclusively medical model of health, since at least, using this model, he can control and shape what medical care or response is delivered. Instead, the doctor should involve himself as an informed citizen in working for those changes and developments which will be productive of health. This would demonstrate and confirm his commitment to health, a good example being the vigorous campaign which doctors have fought against the advertising and sale of cigarettes.

So, I turn now to the second part of the proposed blueprint. My aim here is to identify what action Government could take, using the wide range of institutional mechanisms available to it, but with the NHS and the Department of Health as the central focus for action. That there is a role for Government surely cannot be denied. This is the first point I would emphasize. The present state of our society and, consequently, of the health of the people, is the product of political and economic decisions and circumstances. So, if there is to be any improvement, it will come only through major political, social and economic changes. And for such change, political will and political action are both essential. As Sir George Young, the former Under-Secretary of State at the Department of Health, said recently at a Conference in Stockholm, 'For many of today's medical problems, the answer may not be cure by incision at the operating table, but prevention by decision at the Cabinet table'.

Ironically, Sir George was widely reported as being an early casualty of his own policy. In a Government change he was moved to the Department of Transport, allegedly because of his too energetic attempts to clip the wings of the tobacco industry. Interestingly, Joseph Califano, President Carter's first Secretary of Health, Education and Welfare, brought to his job those very same views on health and, in his autobiography, *Governing America,* also blames the powerful tobacco lobby for his removal from office. It is wise, therefore, to re-emphasize the need for political will. Governments or Ministers, ever aware that theirs is the art of the possible, develop backbone in direct relationship to the degree of popular support they can muster. It behoves us all to raise our voices in the cause of better health.

For my second point, I want to take up Sir George Young's 'decision at the Cabinet table', and consider how it gets translated into policy and action. What is remarkable in the approach of government to the issue of health is the apparent inability, or unwillingness, to see how interrelated are so many of the various decisions of government departments, both national and local. When considering the allocation of resources, it is assumed that claims for spending on, for example, housing or industry or transport or social security compete with claims for spending on health. In fact, of course, they may all be involved in the same exercise.

The point seems obvious. But only recently a junior Treasury Minister said in the House of Commons in answer to a question concerning, as it happens, smoking and revenue, that he was a Treasury Minister, 'not a health Minister'. This is precisely the point. He *is* a health Minister, in that his decisions have a profound impact on health. What leads him to make this statement is, first of all, his failure to understand the social model of health. But equally important is the fact that Government Departments are perceived by those within them as separate compartments. Considerations of health seem to get lost in the scramble by Government Departments for budgets, and the desire for profit or loss in one Department's books, whatever the overall picture. Each Department has its separate brief, its separate interests, its separate policy goals, and, most important, its separate budget. In some senses, each Department is in competition with other Departments. By this reasoning, health comes to be seen as something for the Health Department. Other Departments can then go blithely on making anti-health decisions, arguing spuriously that they are not the Health Department, and leaving the DHSS (and thus the taxpayer) to clear up the mess.

Take the decision of the Minister of Transport in 1977 to approve the restoration of the 70 miles per hour speed limit on motorways. The limit had been reduced to 55 miles per hour at the time of the sudden increases in the cost of oil and petrol in 1973. The decision was taken despite the demonstrable reduction, by 14 per cent, in the number of people killed or injured on the roads between 1973 and 1975. This significant drop was also borne out by evidence from other countries. Some of the reduction may have been due to the fact that cars were used less, because of the increase in petrol prices. But, even allowing for this, the Minister's decision had as an effect the promotion of accidents rather than health. You may well reply that people have to travel by car and need to be able to drive at fast speeds on occasion, and you may add, facetiously, that, on my reasoning, there is a good argument for reducing the speed limit to 5 miles per hour. I concede the need for travel, but would point out that in the United States, where the distances to be travelled are vast by comparison with the United Kingdom, the motorist has been able to live with a 55 miles per hour maximum speed limit. Furthermore, any additional income accruing to the Revenue from increased sales of petrol (as proportionately more petrol is consumed at higher speeds) would undoubtedly be more than offset by the increased costs to the NHS and the Social Services, and thus to the taxpayer, of the increased toll of dead and injured and the needs of their dependants. Such an analysis would demonstrate that, on one calculation, the average taxpayer was being made to subsidize the motorist, whose activity was in fact costing far more than was reflected by the increased price and consumption of petrol. Equally, any rise or fall in the cost, in real terms, of the tax levied on the sale of alcohol will directly affect the numbers of people killed or maimed by drunken drivers.

To take another example, Local Authority spending cut-backs, prompted by loss of national government grants, may well likewise lead to increased spending by national government, if the elderly or disabled have to be admitted to hospital, because the money for such services as home helps, warm meals, social workers, or sheltered housing is no longer there. Decisions in the Industry or the Employment Departments, whether they concern the number of safety inspectors in factories or the level of unemployment, affect directly the promotion or otherwise of health, and consequently the extent of the call on the resources of the Department of Health and Social Security.

Or consider the report in April 1982 from the Government Low Pay

Unit. The number of families caught in the 'poverty trap' had risen from 60,000 in 1979 to 105,000 in 1982. This was solely as a consequence of the decision to alter the level at which income tax is paid. Thus, bizarrely again, decisions to raise revenue merely pile up medical and social security bills for the future. Contrariwise, the Government has spent close to £30 million compensating the victims of byssinosis, but no plans are in hand to offer grants to industry to install new and cleaner machinery or provide better face-masks, although the savings in the future would be great in terms of money and in workers' broken lives.

You would have thought that some properly developed system of co-ordination of policy and spending within Government, aimed at promoting and improving health, would have a very high priority. In fact, such a system seems almost entirely lacking. Some institution-alized mechanism must be created, as a matter of urgency, to provide co-ordination between the various Departments of Government in matters touching on health. Such a body would identify and review measures taken by any particular Department which might have an impact on health. In its role as co-ordinator, it would comment on, criticize, or oppose measures, as the case may be, in the light of the declared function of promoting and improving health. It could occasionally instigate proposals. For example, imaginative proposals to employ financial or tax incentives in efforts to improve or promote health are few and far between. The elderly could be helped to avoid the poverty trap, and its ensuing threat to health, by simple measures such as removing the liability to forfeit social security benefits once earnings rise above a certain sum. The loss of revenue involved would be far outweighed by savings in health and social services spending because of a healthier and happier and more productive elderly population.

Admittedly, the Exchequer has used taxation to some extent as a device to control cigarette consumption, but with considerable ambivalence, given the revenue it derives from the tax on cigarette sales. Remarkably, the cost in real terms of alcoholic beverages has declined in the past decade, despite warnings of an epidemic of alcoholism. Compare the approach by Government in France to one problem, that of infant and maternal mortality rates. These were dramatically reduced, from 22 per cent above the United Kingdom in 1960 to 10 per cent below in 1970, not only because resources were invested in manpower and buildings, but also through the use of such devices as financial benefits made available to pregnant women, conditional upon regular attendance at antenatal clinics. Since the infant mortality rate is a good indicator of child health, it is likely that the proportion of handicapped children in the population is now less in France than in the United Kingdom, with consequent savings to the public purse, let alone the increased happiness among the citizenry.

For my third point, I turn again to health care in the community. I have already referred to the neglected status it has within the system of medical care. Here, I want briefly to draw attention to the way it is organized at governmental level. It is fair to say that such action as there is on the part of Government seems bedevilled by a confusion of aims and complexity of organization. Nowhere is this more true than in the case of the provision made for environmental health. As H.A. Waldron points out, 'The main problem relating to environmental health is . . . the fragmentation of services . . . There is expertise in abundance . . . but it is scattered haphazardly throughout many different organizations and institutions.' As the issues become more complex, the mechanisms for response, through their complexity, become less capable of meeting the need. 'Consider the control of pesticides', Waldron suggests. 'In England no less than nine departments are involved to some degree, in Scotland, three, whilst the Welsh Office protects some of the Welsh interests . . . With so many thumbs in the pie', he concludes, 'it is not difficult to see that the right boy may not always get the plum.'

As a response to this, I would commend to you a proposal which Draper's Unit, in particular, has argued for. This is the creation and use of community health teams at local level. Draper calls for a new public health initiative, a second public health revolution, if you will. Both of these expressions capture perfectly the idea and the spirit behind it; that of building upon the great successes of the nineteenth-century public health movement. Draper sees it as essential, as do I, to look beyond individual-oriented health promotion, towards the creation of teams which will promote health on behalf of the individual; which will, in other words, constitute a structural approach to health promotion, seeking to mould the structure of society, rather than imagining that all can be left to the individual. The public health or community health teams at local level would operate like the old Medical Officer of Health. They would focus on the local community and serve to maximize the adoption of health-enhancing policies, not only at the local level but also at a national level, by making known the circumstances they encounter locally. They would therefore address themselves not only to such matters as fitness or antenatal care, but to transport policy, or ecology, or the environment. Such a scheme, which has been well developed by Draper, offers an exciting opportunity for a Government, whether local or national, with the courage and sense to grasp its significance.

I come now to a series of points the importance of which cannot be overstated. They are at the very heart of this part of the proposed blueprint which is concerned with political action and change. Let me list them in outline first. They involve concern for the poor and the notion of health for all, the role of health education, the need to combat, through Government action, the forces which undermine health, and concern for children.

I will begin with the poor and disadvantaged. We have already seen the obstacles in the way of their access to medical care. What I want now to draw your attention to is a simple proposition. Of all the causes of ill health in our society, relative poverty is the most significant. Thus, if we are to do anything to improve the health of the nation, we must address ourselves to this fact. And, largely, this means that we must look to Government policy. In doing so, we must take note of an argument which, although critically important, may well be overlooked. If health is affected by the sort of forces and factors I have already outlined, some, indeed most of you reading these words, are in a position to pursue them relatively successfully and so, to that extent, can choose to be healthy. We can stop our enquiry at this point. We can say that we have recognized the various determinants of health and can now put ourselves in a position to satisfy them. We, the informed and articulate middle class, have got the message, if you will. And the prevailing political ideology of today would seem to suggest that it would be appropriate to stop at that point. It would seem to suggest that this degree of access to that which promotes our health is all that is possible or even desirable. Knowing is enough. Knowing begets doing. There is abroad, as you well know, a revived infatuation with *laissez-faire*, with what I would describe as Social Darwinism: opportunities abound, let those who can, take them. The rest have only themselves to blame.

The darker side of this particular equation, however, is that the disadvantaged and the less advantaged are losing out. They are less and less able to gain access to these various health-promoting factors. They are losing out whether in terms of relative poverty, jobs, transport facilities, social services and recreational facilities, or in terms of less tangible benefits, such as the enjoyment of parks, visits to football matches or the cinema, the relaxation and diversion offered by holidays, and the peace of domestic harmony, as unemployment, for example, sows its seed of domestic discord and dissolution.

Inequalities in Health, the Black Report, chronicles the awful details. At birth and in the first month of life, the death rate of babies born to parents in social class 5, the unskilled, is double that of babies born to parents in social class 1, professional workers. In the next eleven months, four times as many boys and five times as many girls in class 5 will die, as compared with class 1. Compared with class 1, men in class 5 have twice the rate of long-standing illness, women in class 5 two and a half times the rate. A baby born of social class 1 parents can expect to live five years longer on average than a child of social class 5 parents. If social class 4 (the semi-skilled) and social class 5 had had the same mortality rates as social class 1, in 1970–2 (the latest years for which there are reliable figures) 74,000 people, including 10,000 children, would not have died. Indeed, if a line were drawn from the Wash to the Bristol Channel, those living north of the line, the large majority of whom are members of social classes 4 and 5, have on average a shorter lifespan and higher disease rates than those living south of the line.

The 1979 Report of the Royal Commission on the NHS noted bleakly that in terms of health 'the position of those in social classes 4 and 5 appears to have worsened relative to those in social classes 1 and 2 since the inception of the National Health Service in 1948', though it goes on to point out that all social classes are healthier than thirty years ago. This made the almost contemptuous dismissal of Sir Douglas Black's Report by the then Secretary of State, in a Foreword to the Report, hard to understand. Indeed, every effort was made to minimize the impact of the Report, since, after all, it was commissioned by the previous Government. The number of copies printed was kept to the barest minimum. But such tactics usually contain within them their own nemesis. Once the news of the Report's findings was out, the Report became one of the most photo-copied of all Government documents!

The Secretary of State admitted 'disappointment' that there was generally little sign of health inequalities diminishing. But, he went on, additional expenditure, on the scale which could result from the recommendations of this Report, could be upwards of £2 billion a year. This, he concluded, was quite unrealistic. The cost factor was not argued in the Foreword, nor, it seems, was any account taken for possible short- or long-term savings and benefits which would accrue to a country whose people are healthier. And no account at all was taken of values other than monetary ones, the most obvious being the sheer injustice of operating a system which fails to meet its stated aim, the provision of health care, in its widest meaning, with equality of entitlement and access.

On 31 July 1981, Sir George Young, the then Under Secretary, addressed the issue of cost in reply to a question put to him in Parliament. He said that the cost of implementing the recommendations had gone up to £4,848 million. Again, savings are not considered, in the long and short term. And, even if this figure is accepted, it is, as one Opposition spokesman put it, still considerably less than that committed to the purchase of the Trident missile programme. Sir George then went on to criticize the proposal in the Report that some of the cost be raised by withdrawal of the married man's tax allowance for families without children. 'One could do that,' he replied. 'However, it would mean taking away money from one group and giving it to another. The Government has responsibilities for all members of society. They could not lightly take such a step.' Such reasoning is simply staggering in its hypocrisy. If the Government has responsibility for all members of society, then once a case has been made that some are worse off, a respectable argument exists that the Government's responsibility lies in their doing something extra. Inaction merely confirms the *status quo*, such that Sir George should have said that the Government's responsibility is that all members of society stay where they are. As for taking money away from one group and giving it to another, is this not what taxation is all about? Was it not Sir George's Government which took money in the form of tax from the low paid, who previously paid little or none, so as to make up, in part, the loss of revenue caused by reducing the tax burden of the higher-income earners?

But, in fairness, I may be taking for granted the answer to a question which must be asked and answered. Do we care? Or, do we care enough to see that something is done to remedy, to the extent possible, this state of affairs? If we do not, then we may not see things in terms of injustice, or may regard this as just another of the injustices which afflict mankind, but of as much immediate concern as the odd earthquake in Peru, in response to which the donation of last season's shoes is gesture enough. My concern, however, is health for all, that ringing phrase which the World Health Organization issued as a challenge to the nations of the world in its Declaration of Alma Ata in 1978, when it urged health for all by the year 2000. Article 5 of the Declaration reads, in part, 'Governments have a responsibility for the health of their people which can be fulfilled only by the provision of adequate health and social measures . . . Primary health care is the key to attaining this target as part of development in the spirit of social justice.' Mine is an egalitarian posture. And, quite frankly, I may simply be old-fashioned, out of date, unable to realize that fashions in politics as well as in other things have changed. Indeed, I was quite recently described as a product of '*l'esprit de soixante-huit*', a deliciously pejorative term, suggesting that I had avoided the harsh rite of passage into maturity and was still nostalgically yearning for the students' Utopia broadcast on the streets of Paris and elsewhere in 1968. Despite such strictures, however, I remind those whom I previously described as the middle class, those with greater chances of securing health, that the picture is not all rosy even for them. Although, as I have said, they can to some extent make informed choices about their fate, they are increasingly coming to realize that they too are often powerless to affect decisions concerning their environment – social, economic, political or physical. To cite just one example, the commitment to economic growth which is the central premise of the nation may well, as Draper and his Unit argue, trap them into patterns of ill-health which are beyond their powers to affect.

In sum, then, our concern must be with the whole complex of social, economic and political arrangements in our society. Our aim should be to create an environment more conducive to health for all, to the greatest extent possible, within the political framework, and conceding the necessity, indeed the desirability, of compromise. Put baldly in this way, some of you may say that you have heard enough, and reach for the nearest novel! All this is too big, too grandiose an enterprise, even if it were worth doing in the first place. It is just another in the long line of blueprints for remaking the world! I understand this view. But I do not think we need be so defeatist, though it is right to remain pessimistic. We can, I think, begin to develop some strategies which could edge us towards the desired goal.

One of these strategies is health education. To establish the basis for the promotion and pursuit of health as well as the prevention of illness, there must be a commitment to education. We need, quite simply, to learn how to live healthy lives or, even more fundamentally, we need to have the opportunity to learn. Such education must begin in schools and be carried on in the office, in public forums, in the workplace and in the home. But do not be deceived into thinking that herein lies the answer to the problem. Health education is fine as far as it goes. It does not, however, go all that far. Let me explain. Health education is, by and large, addressed to the individual. But such a strategy is only of limited value. It is flawed in that it assumes that, once informed, the individual will change his behaviour or way of thinking. It overlooks the reality that the individual is, to a very large extent, the product of the social and political environment in which he finds himself, to the extent that knowing something does not necessarily mean that the individual will be able, or indeed sometimes want, to do anything about it. Despite this flaw, exhortations concerning better health addressed to the individual are the basic strategy of the Government-funded Health Education Council and most of the other organizations involved. While I do not discount the fact that they are of some value and can, indeed, be very effective and fruitful, it is a matter of regret that strategies directed at achieving structural change in society, at removing or minimizing the health dangers about which the individual is being educated, and which I shall refer to in a moment, are largely ignored by those involved in health education. The attitude adopted is, in effect, that of saying, 'well, now you know what's good for you, it's up to you to pull your socks up'. Clearly, it is desirable to seek to inform people as individuals. Information is always power, as it offers the evidence on which to plan actions. It may even produce occasionally pressure for structural political change. But it is naive to imagine that the individual inhabits a kind of vacuum in which merely to be informed of what course is the best carries with it the capacity to take that course. This is particularly so when, at the same time, powerful lobbies exist to misinform or manipulate. To take just a couple of examples, it is certainly the case that to live high up in a tower block of flats, in a depressed area, where there is a high incidence of vandalism and crime, is stressful. And stress of that kind undermines good health. But if you live in such a flat, and suffer stress, and have no prospects of moving to other accommodation, it is not entirely clear how this information will help. If anything it could well increase your stress! Equally, there seems to be good evidence that the incidence of suicide increases proportionately with the rate of unemployment among the working population. But if you are unemployed, and also

65

suicidally depressed as a consequence, this particular piece of information is hardly likely to enable you to escape from the unhealthy state you find yourself in. Indeed, the realization that job satisfaction is so important to the maintenance of good health may well depress you further, and exhortations to find a job as the first step to better health might just persuade you to swallow all the sleeping tablets!

Indeed, it is as well to notice that health education can even operate perniciously against improvements in health. Modern medicine has, of course, come to recognize that a large measure of modern illness, not related to genetic disability, is the product of our behaviour and our environment. The main causes of chronic illness and death are heart and respiratory ailments, cancer and strokes, with accidents contributing a large share also. Cigarette smoking, alcohol consumption, appalling dietary habits, dangerous work-places and roads are heavily implicated. Unable to do anything about these conditions, Government and medical men have resorted to the apologia that they cannot do anything until people change. This has been called the syndrome of 'blaming the victim'. For example, the last resort of those faced with the carnage of lung cancer is to say, 'We have done our best. We have shown the link between smoking and cancer of the lung. It is just that people will not stop smoking.' People are castigated as feckless or irresponsible. They eat the wrong foods. They drink too much. Pregnant women will not use the antenatal services available. People just will not take care of themselves. This may appear to let health care and health education off the hook, but what is ignored is the fact that the victim, the one whose life patterns are responsible for his illness, is a product of his environment and often can do little to shape or control it. You can only make the right choices as to food or lifestyle if you have, besides the proper information, the power and capacity to implement your choice.

Having said this, there may, nonetheless, be some circumstances in which changes in individual behaviour or attitudes can be effected through good health education. To the extent that it is possible, it is clearly the task of many groups and institutions and cannot be a matter only for the Health Education Council and like bodies. Government can take the lead through the policies it adopts and the measures it takes, as can industry. It must be said, however, that concern for health has not figured prominently in the actions of industry, if we consider in this respect the question of lead in petrol, the factory farming of animals which subsequently become immobile preparations of hormones and antibiotics, dangerous work-places, or transportation systems which isolate some communities and condemn others to such pollutants as noise and noxious fumes. The motor industry continues to manufacture a class of vehicles designed and advertised in such a way as to invite disaster. But it is the young man who is blamed as feckless or irresponsible when he crashes the overpowered and fragile motorcycle or sports car. In such a case, one answer may lie in Government doing more in the way of controlling advertising standards rather than leaving the regulation of advertising largely in the hands of the advertisers.

Industry and the Trade Unions could make a considerable con-tribution to health if they were to rethink their attitude towards employees' health. At present, most employers still think (if at all) of sick pay or benefit schemes. The financially better-off think in terms of membership of such private medical care schemes as BUPA. Few, if any, think seriously in terms of introducing fitness classes and recreational activities into the working day, rather than as something outside work, or of organizing planning sessions on the prevention of work accidents, again within the working day. I emphasize this point about organizing activities within the work day, since many em-ployers do provide recreational facilities for use out of work. These, of course, tend only to be used by those employees who are already motivated towards maintaining health and fitness. Indeed, Govern-ment could encourage this by requiring that such arrangements be part of the standard contract of employment, or be incorporated into work standards. Tax incentives or interest-free loans could be made available to do whatever building or conversion of premises were necessary or to purchase equipment. But you can almost see the apoplectic industrialist retorting that he runs a factory, not a holiday camp. Such a response typifies much of British industry, with its conservatism and unthinking refusal to countenance change, even if it is urged that it would save money, improve productivity and foster good labour relations. Employers, with the tacit connivance of union leaders, would rather waste money on private medical care which shuts the door after the horse has bolted. Such schemes are, after all, so attractive, selling that sense of self-important status (the private patient) so beloved of the British and gratifying the employer in his sense of *noblesse oblige.*

Another institutional mechanism which could be widely employed is one which has already proved successful in this country and in the

67

United States. It involves the use of members of the affluent middle classes, professionals and such people as entertainers or sportsmen and -women, as role models. After all, this technique has already been shown to be valuable, if it is remembered that it was doctors who led the campaign against smoking and used their professional status and role to influence others. Equally, such health promotion and preventive measures as fitness and reduction in alcohol consumption have been successfully advocated through the use in advertising of those people who ordinarily are identified as fashion-setters and role models. There are signs now that such techniques are being adopted in the United Kingdom through, for example, the use of the English football captain, Kevin Keegan, in a number of health promotion campaigns and the Scottish 1982 World Cup Football Squad in an anti-smoking campaign. Perhaps what is called for is a far more imaginative use of such role models.

Government too has a major role to play in the direction of measures addressed to the individual. The record of succeeding Governments, however, is not good. This is nowhere better illustrated than in the puny budget allocated to the principal agent of Government health promotion, the Health Education Council. Its annual budget is now some £8.5 million. When it is realized that the Council must try to educate us on the dangers of cigarette smoking on about £¾ million, while the tobacco industry spends close to £100 million a year extolling the pleasures of smoking, the extent to which the Council is outfunded and outgunned can be appreciated. The same is true in the case of alcohol, with about £40 million a year being spent by the industry on advertising.

The story is comparable when you consider the case of Health Visitors — nurses who spend a further year of study in preventive medicine. They also have a central role to play, which they discharge with great dedication. But there are too few of them, and, as the Royal Commission on the NHS pointed out, training opportunities are inadequate. Equally, the Commission highlighted the need for more health education officers, whose job it is to promote adult health education. In 1977 there were a mere 300 for the whole of Britain. By 1982 it had risen to just 414. Doctors too have a role to play in this educative process, whether in the surgery or the out-patient department, whether about diet or accidents in the home. But, according to Professor McKeown, it is a major problem to get doctors to think in terms of the community, the environment, preventive care and the promotion of health, as against the diagnosis and treatment of established disease. Lastly, public education can, of course, come through the medium of the press, radio and television. Consider how much attention is given by these to strikes, and even threats of strikes, as imperilling our national well-being through lost working days. I am certainly not saying that strikes should not be reported, and I concede that they can have drastic effects. Over the last decade an average of 13 million working days have been lost each year through strikes. But where is the headline and leader column, the news flash and interview concerning tooth decay, which accounts for an average of 4 million lost working days a year, costs the NHS £200 million a year, and is entirely preventable. Where is the special report on television or in the press on the causes of back pain, which accounts for about 18 million lost working days a year, at a cost to the NHS of £900 million, and which could be greatly reduced through proper education? And where is the outcry in the press against injuries at work, which account for an estimated 48 million lost working days a year? Is it too much to hope that the press will at last discover that one-tenth of all lost working days are the result of bronchitis, which kills 30,000 people a year, costs the NHS several hundred million pounds, as well as lost productivity and social security payments, yet could be greatly reduced if cigarette smoking were curbed? Is it too much to hope that there will be some rethinking in Fleet Street as to what is really 'the English disease'?

Because of the inherent shortcomings of individual-oriented health education, it is clear that more far-reaching action is called for in pursuit of better health. What is needed is for Government not merely to educate us about the risks, but to take on and combat what Professor Morris, in his paper in the *British Medical Journal* of 19 January 1980, called 'the multi-million pound anti-health forces' — the tobacco, alcohol and food industries and their advertisers, who bombard us with misinformation. Government must develop strategies for confronting the threat posed by the major destroyers of our day — cigarettes, alcohol, poor diet and accidents (whether at home, at work or on the road). The attitude of the present Government, however, does not differ greatly from those which have gone before. They are all in favour of preventive measures and health education (after all, who would not be!), but the support seems to stop short of doing anything serious about them. For example, only recently, in the spring of 1982, at a meeting in Southampton, Mr

Finsberg, a Junior Minister in the Health Department, said, when asked about the Government's attitude towards fluoridation of drinking water, that 'virtually all dental problems could be prevented, but we as a Government are not pressing for fluoridation through legislation'. The *laissez-faire* solution, in other words, is the better approach, despite the fact that it means nothing gets done.

Take cigarette smoking first. The Government of the day had its first meeting with the tobacco industry some twenty-three years ago. Yet cigarette advertisements are still all about us. Meanwhile, 1,000 die prematurely each week from the effects of cigarette smoking. About 1,500 babies die each year, and many more are handicapped, because their mothers smoked during pregnancy. Despite the hundreds of millions of pounds spent here and elsewhere in the pursuit of the treatment and cure of lung cancer, in the true traditions of modern scientific medicine, and with little or no success, relatively little work has been carried out by medical researchers (as opposed to advertisers) to discover why people smoke, and how they can be helped to stop. Only in May 1980 the Secretary of State at the DHSS announced in Parliament that his Department was to sponsor research into the motives and pressures causing people, especially the young, to smoke. He expected, he said, that the report would be available by the end of 1981. It has not yet appeared. Why, it could be asked, has it taken so long to commission such research, particularly in view of the increase in cigarette smoking documented by Lesley Doyal in her outstanding book, *The Political Economy of Health*? Between 1958 and 1975 there was an increase in smoking of 9 per cent for men and a startling 63 per cent for women in social class 5, with a consequent increase in death from lung cancer, while in social class 1 there was a fall of 53 per cent for men and 15 per cent for women.

One cause of reluctance to take on the tobacco industry stems, of course, from the tangled economic arguments. It is estimated that between 4 and 5 per cent of government revenue comes from tobacco sales tax. In 1975, *New Scientist* reported that a 'grisly analysis' had been carried out by the Health Department, showing that 'a reduction in smoking would eventually cost the country more than was gained; not only would there be loss of revenue from taxation but also the additional "burden" of having to pay out pensions to the people who had given up smoking before it killed them'. And of course there are about 30,000 jobs in the tobacco industry to consider, not to mention the £11½ million that newspapers derive from advertisements, and the livelihood of corner shopkeepers.

These are the arguments which support the *status quo*. I would make two comments. First, any economic analysis is so extraordinarily hard to carry out that conclusions such as those arrived at by the Health Department must be viewed with great suspicion. Second, there are, of course, values other than money, such as happiness and health, which should not be ignored and which, even in the case of a purely economic analysis, would significantly affect the conclusions arrived at. I hardly need stress that the economic indicator of productivity is much affected by the health and sense of personal satisfaction of the workforce.

It can come as no surprise, however, that the present Government continues the 'hands-off' policy. As the *British Medical Journal* of 14 November 1981 reports, Mr Finsberg, in one of his first speeches on taking office at the Department of Health, said (and this was a speech to the European Ministers Responsible for Public Health, no less), 'My Government does not welcome the use of regulatory or legislative measures in order to control . . . the legitimate commercial freedom of tobacco companies.' At the meeting in Southampton to which I referred earlier, Mr Finsberg was able to advise his less than enthusiastic audience of health-care professionals and educators that, despite the fact that there are now some 50,000 early deaths annually from smoking-related illnesses, the Government would not move to stop cigarette advertising nor ban smoking in public places. 'We live in a free society,' he went on, 'and we do not believe that legislation is the way to do it.' Some may find this a less than convincing argument. Mr Finsberg seemed unembarrassed by the apparent *non sequitur,* ignoring as it does the fact that there are a number of freedoms which are the product of, and are guaranteed by, legislation. As I said at Southampton in response, 'the Government's position is "let them peddle their wares and we will pick up the pieces" '. This position is made all the more difficult to understand by the announcement that, after the most recent round of talks between the tobacco industry and Government, it had been decided to levy a certain sum in the way of tax which would be set aside for health education purposes. Presumably this would include anti-smoking advice!

In the light of such an attitude towards the tobacco industry and the revenue it produces, there seems little hope of any major improvements on this particular front in the war against the anti-health forces. But I insist that certain strategies could still ˙be developed which, even if they do not go the whole way, would make some significant impression on the problem. For instance, the Government could well exclude the tobacco industry from the sponsorship of sport, taking over the role at present played by the industry or encouraging other less socially unworthy sponsors. The former alternative would involve, of course, expenditure, which could be as much as £100m a year, but the savings in the long term to the nation and, therefore, the taxpayer through reduced calls on the Health and Social Security Services would more than compensate for this both financially and spiritually. The money could even come from the existing NHS budget if brave decisions were made concerning the reallocation of money away from certain high-cost medical enterprises, the benefits of which to the general population are at best debatable. The latter alternative could be achieved by such measures as offering appropriately favourable tax exemptions to enterprises not engaged in anti-health activities which were willing to sponsor sport.

Other strategies should include continued pressure for the restriction or banning of smoking in public places. There is a growing trend towards this in the United States and if it were implemented with appropriate vigour in the United Kingdom its effects could be most beneficial. For those who mouth the usual tired arguments about freedom of choice, it is as well to remember that such espousals of individual rights are not unknown in the USA but have been adequately refuted by, for example, reminding the advocate of smoking that the non-smoker may also have some rights. Perhaps the more important strategy involves simply the understanding that resort to tobacco meets a need and that efforts should be made to meet this need less injuriously. Clearly, the reduction of stress is an important effect of smoking. It would be silly to argue that stress can be completely banished from our society. It is quite defensible, however, to urge the development of less dangerous means of dissipating stress.

Then there is our diet. The food industry, as Doyal again ably demonstrates, has been enormously successful in ruining our diet, and consequently our health. For example, more and more food is made from raw materials which have been refined. Look at bread. The ordinary loaf of white bread is not lacking in nutrition. What it lacks is bulk. This lack encourages overconsumption. Overconsumption sells more bread and so produces greater profits. It also produces obesity and a consequent threat to health. And the story has a twist in the tail. The food industry has gone on to develop a second string to its bow, the sale of health foods and vitamin tablets. To make up for what has been removed from some food by its being processed and refined, vitamins and health foods — which are, of course, more expensive than ordinary food — then appear on the market. Thus, the wealthier can get the food they need, since they can afford to buy it. The poor cannot and another inroad into health promotion and the prevention of illness is made. Another example Doyal refers to is the successful campaign to persuade mothers to use modified cow's milk rather than breast-feed their babies. Not only does the baby fail to obtain immunities gained through mother's milk, but mothers are also encouraged to switch from bottle-feeding to commercially prepared solid food as soon as possible, despite the fact that this contributes to child obesity. So successful was the campaign that by the mid-1970s only about 6 per cent of mothers in the United Kingdom breast-fed their babies at 3 months, according to a 1974 DHSS Report. Something like 50 per cent of mothers breast-feed initially, but stop within a relatively short period of time.

As regards accidents, in addition to the 650 killed at work each year, there are a further 6,500 deaths from accidents in the home and at play. Each week 100 miners suffer disabling injuries, yet the occupational health service continues to be neglected. Despite the annual carnage on the roads of about 75,000 people injured and 7,500 killed, only a third of drivers wear safety belts. Furthermore, in the case of children in cars it is estimated that 85 per cent of the deaths and 70 per cent of the injuries would have been prevented if the child had been restrained.

The Parliamentary Secretary at the Ministry of Transport told Parliament on 18 December 1980 that the Health Service would save between £6 million and £7 million a year if seat belts were worn by all front-seat occupants. The taxpayer would be saved a further £10 million a year in social security benefits. And lost productive output which would be saved had, he said, been estimated at £100 million a year. But despite such huge potential savings, around £117 million a year, it was only in 1982 that legislation was finally passed making it compulsory to wear seat belts, with effect from January 1983.

The story of alcohol is similar to that of cigarettes. The Health Education Council spends about £½ million publicizing the health dangers of alcohol, while about £40 million is spent advertising its pleasures by the industry. According to a Report of the Royal College of Physicians, published in March 1980, we are already experiencing an epidemic of alcoholism. Besides causing cirrhosis, the number of deaths from which has doubled to 2,000 a year in the past twenty years, alcohol is also implicated in such illnesses as cancer, heart disease and strokes. Equally, it is linked to the incidence of crime, domestic violence and absenteeism. And, of course, its effect on driving is well known. An estimated 30 per cent of road accident deaths are the result of someone driving while incapable through alcohol. Among young people, it is estimated to be the principal cause of road accident deaths. The immediate preventive effect of the Road Traffic Act 1967, which introduced the breathalyser, was enormous, saving an estimated 1,000 lives in the first year after it became law. But things have become progressively worse. Despite spending by Government of large sums of money (£500,000 in 1977 alone) seeking to persuade drivers not to drink and drive, the problem seems only to be worse. The case is surely made for stronger Government action.

Of course, it is fair to note that there are those who, when faced with the prospect of seat belt legislation, or increased taxes on cigarettes or alcohol, will argue that there is a limit to the extent to which Government should (not can, but should) interfere in the life of the individual. When Chadwick, the pioneer of public health legislation, had his legislation defeated in 1854 and disappeared from public life, *The Times* thundered, 'We prefer to take our chance with cholera, than to be bullied into health'. There is much that is cant and unreason in such calls for individual freedom, even though there is also a perfectly respectable philosophical argument. For, in today's society, there is little an individual can do which does not impinge on others. The smoker, for example, draws sickness pay, receives medical care and dies in hospital, all funded from public revenue. When he cannot work, he and his dependants are supported from public funds. Equally, the driver or passenger who fails to wear his seat belt is treated in the intensive care unit and recuperates in hospital at a high cost to the public purse. And if he dies or cannot work he and his family live off public funds.

Let us consider next two other threats to health, often overlooked. They are unemployment and the level of subsistence available to those who must rely on social security benefits. Unemployment has of course a number of devasting effects, not least the loss of a sense of worth and consequent desperation or frustration. Unemployment also threatens health in the sense that family income and consequent levels of nutrition and quality of housing and recreation are affected adversely. Harvey Brenner, in a now famous study at Johns Hopkins University in the United States, has shown that the increase in unemployment in the United States between 1970 and 1975 of 1¼ million people was responsible for an extra 26,000 deaths from heart and kidney disease, 5,500 extra admissions to mental hospitals, 1,700 extra homicides, 1,500 extra suicides and 900 extra deaths from cirrhosis, through excessive consumption of alcohol. Studies in Australia and here in the United Kingdom bear out this thesis, though, not surprisingly, this work is not without its critics. Malcolm Colledge, in his thoughtful review in 1981 of the research, *Unemployment and Health,* concludes that, 'a reduction in the general level of economic activity triggers off a sequence of events which result ultimately in increased levels of ill-health and death rates'. The principal reasons for this, he argues, 'lie in increased levels of stress on individuals. This stress is caused by social pressures, financial difficulties, family and marital relationships, a disruption of daily patterns, a challenge to the ingrained work ethic. The response to this stress varies with personality and socio-economic position, but there is a significant number of cases where the result is ill-health in one form or another.' Furthermore, as a task force of the United States Department of Health, Education, and Welfare reported in 1973, 'in an impressive 15-year study of ageing, the strongest predictor of longevity was work satisfaction'. Such arguments lend a cutting edge to the polite political debate about the regrettable level of un-employment.

Equally, those who live on social security benefits constantly teeter on the brink of ill health. As *The Times* of 22 January 1982 reported, unemployment benefit has now been reduced to its 1951 level com-pared with wages. Already, many of the elderly and disabled live in a state of relative poverty. Already, many of them have difficulty in meeting the costs of keeping warm in winter, living as they do in substandard housing. And with the cold comes ill health and, to some, death. Limit further the resources available to them and the risks only grow. Already, many are socially isolated and subsist on the barest minimum of food. With malnutrition comes ill health and, to some, death. Limit further the resources available and the risks only grow.

Of all the points in this blueprint for better health, I have left the most important until last. Not only does it provide a suitable con-clusion, but it ties together many of the themes about medical care and health which I have already considered. I refer to the health of our children. If we are to improve the health of the nation, we have no choice but to redirect an enormous amount of our resources to the care of children, before birth, at birth, and during their development. If ever there was a case for the promotion of health, this must be it. It is in fact one of the declared priorities of the NHS, but little yet has been achieved. Indeed the results are disgraceful. Once again, it has to be realized that what is needed is not just a tinkering with or retooling of the NHS. The result would be cosmetic at best. What is called for is the realization that the state of our children's health and, thus, their and our future is a consequence of the whole style of our society and that if anything is to be done, then some fairly profound political action is called for.

It is a measured understatement to say that as a society we could do more for the health of our children. The problem of course is not new. As Muir Gray points out, the improvement in the general health of adults at the end of the nineteenth century was not accompanied by improvements in child health. So low was the level of fitness of the British working class that half the young men who volunteered for the Boer War were turned away as unfit. The minimum height for entry into the infantry had to be dropped from 5 feet 6 inches in 1882 to 5 feet in 1902. The shock was such as to provoke the passing of legislation in 1906 and 1907 to establish a school medical and school meal service. The thinking was not, of course, wholly philanthropic or egalitarian. There was also a need for a fitter, more productive labour force.

Our perinatal mortality and morbidity rates in the United Kingdom, the death and sickness rates, compare unfavourably with most other countries of similar economic and social development. And who are the children who are suffering? Let me remind you of the words of Sir Douglas Black's Report, *Inequalities in Health:*

'From the end of the first month to the end of the first year . . . for the death of every 1 male infant in class 1, we can expect . . . 4 deaths in class 5. Among female infants these ratios are even more disadvantageous to the offspring of manual workers.'

Perinatal mortality, death of a baby at birth or in the first week of life, accounts for seven babies per thousand in social class 1, but 27 in every thousand born into social class 5. Antenatal and perinatal care simply are not being delivered to those most in need, those in social classes 4 and 5. Women in these groups, according to Muir Gray, 'go to clinic for the first time later in the course of pregnancy, attend less regularly, and follow the advice given less punctiliously. For instance, they more frequently continue to smoke.' The reasons are many and include, for example, transport difficulties, the siting of clinics, the need to care for other children, an acquired antipathy to authority, and the middle-class attitudes of doctors, with their emphasis on rationality and planning, not shared by the working class. *The Times* of 15 April 1980 carried the report of the Central Birmingham Community Health Council which highlighted the fact that women most at risk in pregnancy came from the poorest homes and had the least adequate facilities available to them. Indeed, the report showed that in inner-city areas, such as Sparkbrook, the perinatal mortality rate was 80 per cent higher than the national average. A second study by the West Midland Regional Health Authority, reported in *The Times* on 6 May 1980, showed that only 21 per cent of pregnant women over forty years of age in this area had recourse to antenatal care, despite their high-risk category.

It is the children of these same families who are no longer immunized against the common infections. Large numbers of parents have, for example, been frightened off by the well-meaning but ill-advised campaign against whooping-cough vaccination. Whereas 80 per cent of children at risk were vaccinated in the early 1970s, only 40 per cent were in 1980. The allegation was that vaccination carried a risk of inducing brain damage in the child. The cause of children who, it was said, had suffered such damage was championed by certain Members of Parliament and the children ultimately received compensation from the State. The proof was not strong, the numbers were very few as compared with the millions who benefited without ill effect, but the cause was popular. The unhappy consequence has been that the attention the campaign attracted caused many mothers to lose confidence in all forms of immunization for their children, not just against whooping cough. Since then, the United Kingdom has seen a mild epidemic of whooping cough in 1978 with some few deaths recorded. Again, in August 1982, another 'big outbreak' was reported by the Communicable Disease Surveillance Centre. It may well be that we shall have to undergo the horrors of a polio epidemic before parents will be persuaded once again to avail themselves of this most basic and easily available of preventive measures.

It is these same children in social classes 4 and 5 who do not receive adequate testing for hearing and sight and whose prospects for educational and emotional development, never the brightest, are handicapped still further. Indeed, the poor services available for the deaf mean that more than half of the children born deaf are not diagnosed until they are at least three years old. Nonetheless, *The Times* of 6 May 1980 reported that, according to the National Deaf Children's Society, teaching services for the deaf were to be cut further by more than a fifth.

It is these same children whose nutrition and health are most affected by political decisions, made in the name of economy, to raise the price of school meals or abandon the service, to curtail the supply of free school milk, to reduce a whole range of social security benefits, whether supplementary benefits or child benefits or even allowances for children's clothing and shoes, to limit access to free school transport, or even dispense with the services and safety afforded by those guardians of the road crossings near schools, the 'lollipop ladies'. Recall, if you will, that about 5,000 children are killed or injured each year while crossing the road, to the extent that Britain has the worst child pedestrian injury rate in Western Europe.

It is these same children who must live in substandard housing. It is these same children who provide the squalid statistic which has it that 97 per cent of them by the age of 15 will have rotting teeth. Fluoridation of drinking water which, it has been estimated, would reduce the incidence of dental caries by a half, continues to attract opposition. You will recall that the present Government is 'not pressing' for legislation. The Royal Commission on the NHS was moved to conclude that 'it is entirely wrong to deprive the most vulnerable section of the population of such an important public health measure, for the sake of the views of a small minority of adults for whom its benefits come too late'. But, quite apart from this, the system of dental care negotiated in 1948 at the outset of the NHS makes little or no provision for preventive dentistry. Nor does the elaborate piece-work system of payment encourage it. As Professor Miller puts it, in his book *Medicine and Society*, 'the financial basis of professional remuneration might have been specifically designed to produce a cheap and nasty service'.

It is these same children who feel the cold wind of unemployment blowing through their parents' lives. It is these same children who will suffer from a mortality rate from accidents five times higher than that of children born into social class 1. In sum, the National Child Development Study, which has followed the development of 10,000 children born in the first week of March 1958, demonstrates, in the words of Muir Gray, that the 'socially handicapped were shorter in height, more often absent from school, more frequently had hearing loss, more often had a squint, and were twice as likely to have had tuberculosis, meningitis or rheumatic fever. Their housing conditions made . . . the spread of infections more probable.' Finally, he notes, 'Not surprisingly, the educational achievement of deprived children was lower. One in fourteen of the disadvantaged children was receiving, or waiting to receive, special education compared with one in eighty of those not socially handicapped and educational subnormality was seven times more common.'

These inequalities, or iniquities, cannot be shrugged off, yet successive governments seem oblivious. The extent of the re-examination and reorientation of values called for is breathtaking. But so also is the extent of the human wastage and misery, which we tolerate now with hardly a thought as to whether things might be otherwise. By contrast to the magnitude of this task, the squabbling over private medicine, which seems to mesmerize politicians and doctors, is a tragic irrelevance. The Black Report observed that 'early childhood is the period of life at which intervention could most hopefully break the continuing association between health and class'. Thus, the Report concluded that 'the abolition of child poverty should be adopted as a national goal for the 1980s'. You will recall the then Secretary of State's thoroughly anaemic comment that the findings of the Black Report on Inequalities in Health will 'come as a disappointment to many'. They are a disgrace; an indictment of what we are and what we have achieved. More than 100 years ago Disraeli spoke of our being two nations. We still have not escaped this indictment. Now let those who want to argue about heart transplants do so. It is against this background that the debate must be judged.

In these brief comments, I have sought to sketch the outline of a programme to improve our health. You may rest assured that those who would oppose it will find reasons of cost to justify doing so. I have little patience with such people. They hide their political choices behind slide rules and balance sheets. My political choices have been made clear. But they are not mine alone. They are what this country purports to stand for. If you begin with them, the figures can come out quite differently.

The strategy must be to press for those kinds of structural change in society which will enhance the health of all. The key must be to make clear how the existing structure militates against health and how, if securing health for society at large is, indeed, a primary goal of any civilized nation, such changes should be made. Central to such an argument is the thesis that improvements in the health of all can only redound to the benefit of the society, whatever aspect of its life is considered. Argument, debate, pressure, all have their place for all those who believe in the power of ideas and of persuasion. We must all constantly argue the case. We must all, of course, live with the realities of compromise. It would be wrong, furthermore, as well as naive, to expect that Government can produce, or set in train, some Utopia of flowing health. But we can demand that as individuals we get a better deal in terms of particular policies or decisions. There is, for example, strong evidence that the 'Great Society' legislation in the United States in the mid-1960s, conceived by President Johnson, significantly improved the health of the less well off and, therefore, of the nation. In their book, *Despite the Welfare State*, Muriel Brown and Nicola Madge suggest the same is possible in the United Kingdom. But, they write, 'it is necessary to reassert the reality of the whole class-related pattern of disadvantage'. Nonetheless, they argue, 'alternative structures are possible, and it is necessary to reassert the potential for a different and better society'. Their work is the result of ten years of study, commissioned by Sir Keith Joseph, then Secretary of State at the DHSS, of what he called the 'cycle of deprivation'. This authoritative and comprehensive study shows that 'the poor are always with us from one generation to the next because the state does not provide enough in the way of housing, schooling, hospital beds or income support', in the words of *The Times* review of 13 July 1982. Such a finding lends support to my argument, though it will not endear itself to the man who commissioned it or to the Government of which he is still part. My message is that progress can be made, albeit interstitially, provided the goal is perceived as limited, and workable proposals are made.

What I have offered is a conceptual framework, a blueprint. It calls for action. If we are to change the way medicine and health are thought of and practised, it is we, through Government, who must take that action. It is our responsibility.

4 'Decisions, decisions . . .'

In practising medicine doctors routinely make decisions, they make judgements. This much is commonplace. But what sort of judgements or decisions are they? All professionals make judgements. That is what we expect of them. That is what we consult them for. 'Leave it to doctor' is an expression which is part of our language, as are such phrases as 'doctor's orders' or 'doctor knows best'. They have, perhaps, been incorporated into our vocabulary without much thought. What are the implications of such language? When we think of doctors' decisions, we think of diagnosis, prognosis, treatment. We think of these decisions as being bounded by and derived from demonstrable objective principles, something called medical expertise. We think of these decisions as matters of medical technical skill, a skill acquired at medical school and deriving from a study of medical science. That is what the doctor goes to medical school for, and then spends years on the job learning about. We call these decisions, medical decisions. This is what doctors have a special, indeed unique, competence in. But are they matters of technical skill? Do these demonstrable objective principles exist? If so, what are they? What is a medical decision? What is this medical expertise? These may appear to be simple enough questions. But the answers are not so simple, even though they go to the heart of the practice of medicine. Define the nature of a medical decision and you define the role played by doctors.

We could define a medical decision by saying it is one taken by doctors. This cannot be right. The decision as to what vote to cast in a general election is made by doctors, but that does not make it a medical decision. So can we narrow the inquiry down a little? Can we say it is a decision made by a doctor in a medical context? No, this will not do either. It is circular: what is medical is what is medical. Let us try another approach. Let us say that, in the most general sense, the doctor claims unique competence in making decisions about health and ill health, illness and disease, and appropriate forms of response, whether treatment or non-treatment. That is the doctor's *raison d'être*, and it is one accepted by the rest of us. This may satisfy some, but it does not satisfy me. First, we have already come to understand that health and illness are not matters of objective reality, on which we all agree, as are, for example, the questions whether humans, generally, have two arms and two legs and one head. Instead, health is a socially determined and evaluative term, just as is its counterpart, ill health. Equally, we have seen that illness is a status — something conferred on someone in the light of particular facts, but not inherent in those facts. The issue is not whether X, objectively, is ill, but whether he ought to be regarded as ill, whether he satisfies certain conditions, which, admittedly, usually include physical realities such as fever or pain (though in the case of mental illness even this requirement is dispensed with), but which also include social, moral and political components, which fail to be considered.

Secondly, the word treatment deserves careful scrutiny. It too is redolent with moral and social assumptions and implications. What makes some responses to a person's problem treatment, while other responses are not so described? I ask this because, of course, the word treatment endows what is done with a certain legitimacy. It is proper, therefore, to be alert to the proper limits of its use. If, for example, a doctor wishes to prescribe heroin or LSD in cases of depression, or wishes to subject a sexually aggressive male to chemical castration, can such prescriptions be called treatments and so gain some sort of moral respectability? Or, to take an example which has provoked considerable controversy in the United States, if a doctor wishes to employ 'sex counsellors' for people encountering so-called sexual dysfunction, is this treatment acceptable because a doctor advised it, or does it remain prostitution, such that the doctor, if he charges a fee for his advice, is living off immoral earnings? Clearly, the distinction is important. Equally clearly, any proposed response or intervention by a doctor must be shown not to offend the laws or moral values of the society. The fact that a particular doctor, or even doctors in general, advocate it and seek to legitimize it by calling it treatment is not enough. We as a society, through our laws and moral code, reserve the right to question the appropriateness and worth of such responses. Merely to call something treatment will not lend it any moral *laissez-passer*. Doctors do not have some sort of moral *carte blanche*. So, once again, factors other than those of a medical-scientific nature have to be weighed.

Some of you may protest that this is a caricature, a travesty of the truth. Yes, you may say, doctors certainly make decisions all the time and these do involve judgements, for example, how to manage a particular patient. 'Manage' is obviously a term involving choices, but, you say, these choices are made by reference to sound medical principles, and out of concern for the patient's best interests. But this still fudges the issue. You still have to tell me what sound medical principles are, and by whom they were developed. You see, my point is that the scope of the alleged unique competence of the doctor is as wide, as imprecise, as flexible and as inherently evaluative as the meanings given to the notions of health, ill health and treatment. Doctors make decisions as to what ought to be done. Some, but only some, of these decisions are matters of technical skill. I submit that the majority of decisions taken by doctors are not technical. They are, instead, moral and ethical. They are decisions about what ought to be done, in the light of certain values. Now, this creates a problem. Doctors claim a special, indeed unique, competence in a particular area, the practice of medicine. So medical judgements, medical decisions, are for them and them alone. But, if I am right that it is a fundamental feature of medical practice that doctors are making ethical judgements, it means that ethics, to the extent that they touch on how doctors choose to practise medicine, are something for them, and them alone. This is a surprising and even dangerous notion.

It would normally be accepted that ethical principles, the principles by reference to which we organize our lives and decide what we ought or ought not to do, are not the preserve of any one group. But the doctor may reply that, yes, he does make ethical decisions, but these are medical ethics, and so they are properly for doctors alone. This would suggest that there is a realm of ethics unique to medicine and within the unique competence of doctors to determine and apply. It would suggest that, by the use of the adjective 'medical', the doctor can define out of competence all those who would otherwise presume to comment on his conduct. It would suggest that the doctor can have recourse to that word so beloved of all professionals, and dismiss commentators as 'laymen'. My response is that medical ethics are not separate from, but part of, the general moral and ethical order by which we live. All that the word 'medical' adds is to indicate that, here, we are talking of ethics in the context of medicine. To argue otherwise is to suggest that business ethics is exclusively the prerogative of businessmen, or legal ethics that of lawyers. Heaven preserve us from either conclusion!

Let me make my point crystal clear. Of course, in one sense, the decisions to be made are for doctors alone to make. They are on the spot, 'in the trenches', as it were. I am not suggesting that others should make them. But the decisions must conform to standards set or agreed upon by others. They must be based on principles. Decisions as to what the doctor ought to do must, in short, be tested against the ethical principles of the society. He has no special dispensation to depart from our moral and ethical order. The only special feature of his particular code of ethics can be the obligation to adhere even more strictly than the average citizen to our ethical order, because of the position of power he occupies.

To many of you, what I have said so far is commonplace. The difficulty is that many doctors in the United Kingdom have been slow, very slow, in accepting it. By contrast, in the United States medical ethics has long passed the point of having to establish its right to exist as a separate field of enquiry. Those working in the field, whether doctor, moral philosopher, theologian, or lawyer, have got down to the job of finding answers to hard problems. Medical opposition has become more and more isolated. Here, however, there is a long way to go. And too often, the moment this debate is opened the floodgates of vitriol are opened also. But the debate should be opened. It must be wrong that power and responsibility in many areas of human concern should be pushed on to doctors by the simple tactic of calling them medical matters, just because we are happy to have others bear this responsibility. Equally, it must be wrong that a doctor, simply by describing a decision as medical, can claim unique competence, and the power which goes with it, to make such a decision, even if it touches the basic values by which we live our lives. For if doctors claim unique competence it must be in something they are uniquely competent to do. Doctors are not uniquely competent to make ethical decisions. They receive no training to prepare them for such a role. They have no preparation in moral philosophy, they have no special skill in ethical analysis. So, put rather bluntly, what I am calling for is a wholesale re-examination of the sphere of alleged competence of the doctor.

If you agree with me, as I take you through some examples, that doctors are indeed making ethical decisions in a rather haphazard, idiosyncratic way, then you will want to consider how best we should respond. We may seek to insist, by whatever means is deemed appropriate, that doctors conform to standards and principles set down by all of us. We may suggest that the education of doctors should prepare them more appropriately for the decisions they are called on to make. We may be content merely to remind them that they must look over their shoulders from time to time, to make sure we approve of what they are doing. I will offer you my views on the proper way to resolve the problems I pose, and on the steps we can take to put our medical ethics into good shape and develop good medical ethics. Some doctors, I am sure, will recognize the truth in what I am suggesting. It is just that they seem to operate on some form of automatic pilot when it comes to matters of ethics. We must gain their attention and provide the correct navigation.

There are others, however, who will take more persuading. After all, doctors did not win their dominance in the field of medicine and healing without a struggle; and, having won it, and the power which goes with it, only with the greatest reluctance will an inch of ground be conceded. Not much more than 100 years ago, those whom we now call doctors competed with many others in the market place of the healing arts. Gradually, scientific medicine won the day in Europe and America. Doctors who chose this new route were licensed and organized themselves into a profession. From such a position of consolidated power, other methods of treating people, other approaches to caring and healing can be denigrated and ostracized as quackery, not only ill conceived, but wrong and possibly harmful. The term 'fringe medicine' is used as if there were a central core of proper medical care. Indeed, one of the most interesting social and political conflicts of the next decade will be the challenge of this view.

I want now to look at some particular ethical problems, by way of illustrating the general theme. You will see what they involve and how they are customarily solved. I will also offer my analysis. Having done this, having jumped in at the deep end, having seen how easy it is to sink, we can then climb out and stand back to take a more general look at medical ethics. Our aim should be to find a better way of proceeding in the future.

Take the following propositions. You would not, for example, consider the law of homicide, and exceptions to it, to be a matter for doctors alone to decide upon. Nor would you regard it proper for doctors alone to decide when principles of honesty should be observed or waived. Nor would you regard it proper for doctors alone to decide the appropriate conditions of family life. These are all examples of social and political decisions which go to the root of our culture. Would it surprise you, then, to learn that each is an example of a decision commonly taken by doctors, and regarded as uniquely within their competence to make? And, if it is uniquely within their competence, it follows that only doctors, and no one else, may properly challenge such a decision.

It is doctors who decide whether or not to treat a baby born severely handicapped. And notice, I am not talking here of a baby who is so ill that he will die inevitably, come what may. In such a case, the doctor clearly only has a duty to make the death as comfortable as possible. The baby I am considering will not die if it receives the care which babies are ordinarily given. But it will not prosper. It will always be severely handicapped. It may be suffering from Down's Syndrome — what used to be called mongolism — or from spina bifida, a condition which, in its severest form, is attended by gross paralysis of the limbs, incontinence, the accumulation of fluid in the brain and the possibility (which cannot be accurately predicted) of the severest mental handicap.

Let us consider the fate of this spina bifida baby. The question posed is what to do. The fluid on the brain can be controlled, and, with a lengthy succession of careful surgical operations, some of the worst deformities may be corrected, although function lost cannot be restored. Should this treatment be embarked upon? Perhaps it is as well to know that if it is not, the baby will more than probably die, usually by recourse to what can best be described as benign neglect. The baby may be fed only on demand, while given sedatives which suppress demand. Or the baby may be nursed, but allowed to succumb to the first infection without recourse to appropriate medications. An awesome decision therefore falls to be made. And who makes it? It is the doctor who makes it. It has to be. He is the one charged with the care of the baby. Very often, the parents will be involved, but I put it to you that this involvement should not be regarded as significant in terms of the nature of the decision arrived at, though it may be important in the process of decision making. This is because parents tend to do what doctors advise. Even if the doctor purports not to advise, but merely to state the facts neutrally, nothing is changed, for it is clear that the choice as to which facts to present and how to present them will produce the same result as that produced by more direct advice.

On what criteria does the doctor decide? This is what concerns us here. We have seen that the decision is the doctor's, but that the principles guiding him are not. There are probably many. One criterion may be his view as to the proper allocation of resources within the finite amount available to him or, more generally, to the NHS as a whole. Another may be the wishes of the parents. Perhaps the principal criterion relied upon is one called the quality of life. From observation of the common fate of children who, though very severely handicapped, have undergone the most active surgical intervention and treatment, it has been concluded by many paediatricians that the children's lives are just not worth living. Multiple operations and the accompanying pain and distress to child, parent and nursing staff produce little improvement in the child's condition. It remains paralysed, incontinent, and often mentally disabled. Indeed, the history of treatment in England has been one of a shift away from a policy of active surgical intervention to a policy of selective treatment. Only those babies are treated who, on this criterion of the quality of their life, are worth salvaging. The others, as I suggested, usually die, as they did before active intervention was developed in the late 1950s. Indeed, it is an interesting insight into the practices of doctors in this field that, when active intervention was first introduced on a large scale, the number of still births reported to the Registrar General actually declined, suggesting that some, at least, previously included in that number were not genuine still births, but were children encouraged to die after the extent of their handicap was discovered. Also it is of interest to note that, by contrast, certain other countries, particularly Sweden, continue actively to treat a far greater proportion of babies than are treated in England, simply because the social services and institutionalized care available are so much better than in England, such that, once out of hospital, the baby's fate will not be one of distressing neglect despite the love and care of parents.

Now, let us analyse this process objectively. We must first note that the notion that there is a specific quality of life which a baby, unable to speak for itself, would not wish to have, because it falls too far below (however far that may be) what we healthy people conceive as the norm, can hardly be described as scientific. It is self-evidently an evaluation based at best on felt but unarticulated criteria. There is no mechanic's manual, no technician's guide, which indicates when treatment is justified. The doctor decides on the basis of some rough and ready calculus of the baby's future quality of life. And I use the cliché 'rough and ready' because it captures the quality of the doctor's decision, a decision by rote, which has become a stereotype without need for deliberation. Furthermore, it varies with the doctor. There is no agreed course of action, even among doctors. In figurative terms, the baby in Huddersfield lives while the one in Halifax dies.

Can anyone doubt that the principles, by reference to which this enormously profound moral decision is made, as to who should live and die, cannot be left to doctors alone, or even to parents. Doctors have no greater moral insight, or powers of analysis, than the rest of us, so as to claim unique competence to lay down these principles. This seems so clear that you would think opposing views would be impossible. Yet, in fact, to make the point is to attract the odium and hostility of doctors in the field, who are convinced, with a sort of Messianic fervour, of the rightness of their decisions. But I persist. It is not necessarily that I disapprove of what is being done. It may be that we all, or most of us, do approve. What I find utterly objectionable is the notion that this so profound a question is rightfully for doctors alone to decide upon, so that others intrude at their peril. And it is made more objectionable by the fact that, if one is for a moment to play the lawyer, there is at least some suspicion, if not downright certainty, that the law of homicide is having its tail twisted. This would not be the first time we have decided to turn a blind eye. But we should all be given the chance to know and to decide, on the basis of clearly articulated and agreed-upon ethical principles. The doctor overreaches himself in his claim for unique competence.

Nor is this ethical dilemma, captured in the deceptively simple phrase, the quality of life, limited to new-born babies. It arises, for example, each time the doctor decides whether or not to try to resuscitate the person who has attempted suicide. It arises each time a doctor must decide whether a patient dying from kidney failure should receive dialysis treatment or be selected for a kidney transplant. It is an illusion to imagine that the decision will be unaffected by considerations of the 'social worth' of the patient. In the absence of any effective review of the decision, or any established principles, it will be the doctor's view which will prevail, however idiosyncratic. It arises each time the doctor weighs up what to do about his elderly patient who lies paralysed from his latest stroke and now has pneumonia. Should he treat the pneumonia, so that the patient may live another couple of weeks or months? Or should he let the pneumonia be the old man's friend, as it used to be?

Not surprisingly, such dilemmas as these have been brought before the courts in the United States. For several reasons, the courts play a far more active role in the United States than in the United Kingdom in resolving issues of this nature. Two of the most famous recent decisions have been in the Saikewicz case in 1977 and the Quinlan case in 1976. In Saikewicz, Judge Liacos, in the Massachusetts Supreme Court, decided that the question whether a severely mentally retarded man of sixty-seven should receive chemotherapy which would temporarily postpone his death from leukaemia was not one to be decided by doctors alone. The courts must be involved. In their role as guardians of the rights and liberties of each citizen, the courts must be the ones to lay down the principles on which such a decision was to be based. The decision provoked screams of outrage from the medical profession. Arnold Relman, the editor of the *New England Journal of Medicine*, led the onslaught, condemning the decision as a vote of 'no confidence in the medical profession'. The thrust of the critics' argument was that, in the words of R. Reiss, writing in the *Journal of Medical Ethics* of June 1980, 'It seems to us that the experienced physician is in a much better position to make such judgements than either the family or a court of law.'

It seems to me, however, that there are two issues which the critics confuse. First, it must be clear beyond peradventure that a decision such as the one involved in the Saikewicz case, though it must be made by doctors, cannot be made by reference to principles laid down only by doctors, far less the view of one doctor. It must be made by reference to socially established and institutionalized principles. The second issue is the question of who should lay down these principles. Arguably, in the United States the courts are the appropriate agency, *faute de mieux*. In England the courts play a less prominent role and are not seen, as they are in the United States, as the great unifier in an otherwise heterogeneous country. The courts may not, in my view, be the most appropriate agency to lay down the principles in England, although, as we shall see in a moment, there has been a recent flurry of court cases. But, whoever lays them down, the first point remains intact, whether in the United States or England.

The Quinlan case is well known. The parents of Karen Quinlan, a deeply religious couple, petitioned the court for permission to have her cared for without recourse to artificial ventilation. This was thought to be a merciful and morally right course to take. Tragically, she had suffered irreparable brain damage and was in a permanent vegetative state. It was thought that she would die once the ventilator was disconnected. In the event, she did not, and still lies in a New Jersey hospital. The case is undoubtedly exceedingly important for what it decided: that there comes a point beyond which a doctor is no longer under a duty, morally or legally, to persist with forms of treatment which can be described as heroic or pointless. It is equally important because the New Jersey Supreme Court made it clear that such a decision was of such profound philosophical significance that it was for the court, representing the distillation of society's wisdom, not for doctors, to make. On these points at least, the decision was, and has been regarded as, a major advance in the development of humane and sensitive medical law.

This does not stop some, such as Lord Smith, Past-President of the Royal Society of Medicine, from arguing in the same issue of the *Journal of Medical Ethics* that 'the wise and humane physician, in tune with his patient, will know very well when it is time to withdraw treatment. This decision must be made by, and the responsibility borne by, one doctor who has earned and enjoys the confidence and trust of the patient and his family. We must not allow this to become a committee matter. Still less must a decision of this kind become a matter for the courts of law. We have seen, much publicized in the Karen Ann Quinlan case, what happens when an attempt is made to invoke the legal code, and the spectacle was hardly edifying.'

Lord Smith's view must be wrong. Such decisions simply are not to be made on the basis of a particular doctor's wisdom or humanity, great though these may be. Further, to refer to allowing this to 'become a committee matter' is to repeat the confusion I have just pointed out, between the decision as to what to do in a particular case and the decision as to what principles must be followed. This second decision is pre-eminently a matter for some committee, representative body, or other appropriate agency, the nature and composition of which I will return to later. And to denigrate the Quinlan decision is to fail to understand the splendid use of the natural law principles of freedom and privacy, as found in the United States Constitution. It ignores the power for good the decision has become in the United States, not only in its specific detail but also in its embracing a notion that there is a limit to how far massive and pointless medical intervention should be tolerated.

As I said, there has suddenly been a flurry of court cases involving the kind of issues I am discussing. This is an unusual development. Cases involving medical ethical issues are few and far between. It may reflect the lack of clarity felt by many about what conduct is ethically and legally justified, and the need for guidance. It may also reflect the increased visibility of medical ethical problems: the more people become aware of their existence and their complexity, the less they can be resolved by private arrangement. *R* v *Arthur*, decided in November 1981, was concerned with the treatment of a new-born baby with Down's Syndrome as was *Re B* (a minor). *R* v *Reed*, decided in October 1981, was concerned with euthanasia. Because of their very considerable importance, I want to consider them at length, even if this means taking you into greater detail than I have done so far. They provoked a great deal of public attention. There was much debate on the issues they raised, the answers arrived at and the appropriateness of the courts as the medium for deciding. In the long run, this debate can only be a good thing, even if, at the time, not all the debate is informed or considered. It may be that more heat than light is often generated. I am convinced, however, that it is wrong to leave questions concerning, for example, the treatment and future existence of a child to be solved in private, behind closed doors. Painful as it may be, we have to turn over this particular stone and examine what is underneath.

Dr Arthur was acquitted on 5 November 1981 of the attempted murder of a three-day-old baby boy with Down's Syndrome. Dr Arthur had consulted the baby's parents. They had indicated that, given his handicap, they did not wish him to survive. Dr Arthur then prescribed a sedative drug DF 118 which also suppresses appetite, and otherwise ordered 'nursing care only'. The baby died within sixty-nine hours of birth. The defence to the charge was that once the baby's disability was known, Dr Arthur had engaged in a 'holding operation', keeping the baby comfortable and nursing the baby, but otherwise waiting to see whether he would rally and live, or whether 'nature would take its course'. This, it was said, was proper conduct, both ethically and legally.

Does the case give us good law and good medical ethics? I think that if it is understood properly, and the passion and drama of the trial are put aside, it can be seen as edging us towards a position as regards the new-born which is ethically defensible though something of a departure from traditional legal thinking at least, if not from practice.

Let me explain. At first blush, it could be said that the case tells us nothing except that a jury was unwilling to convict a much-respected doctor of a very serious crime. And this would tend to reinforce the view that prosecutions of doctors, with all the hullabaloo which surrounds them, are most inappropriate for shaping medical law and ethics. But the jury had to be instructed as to the law on which to base their finding of fact. So, study those instructions and you get a statement of the legal and ethical duty of the doctor to the handicapped new-born in his charge, as understood by the judge. In my view, Mr Justice Farquharson developed new law in his instructions. He attempted to reshape the law of murder so as to make it sensitive to the moral complexities of modern medicine. He did not do it particularly clearly, nor was his analysis all that sound. But he did provide something to build on so as to develop good medical law and ethics.

In his instructions to the jury, Mr Justice Farquharson indicated that it was lawful to treat a baby with a sedating drug and offer no further care by way of food or drugs or surgery if certain criteria were met. These criteria appear to be, first, that the child must be 'irreversibly disabled' and, second, 'rejected by its parents'. By way of clarification for the jury, the judge drew a distinction between sedating the baby and passively letting it die, 'allowing nature to take its course', and doing a positive act to kill the baby — for example, giving it a death-dealing dose of drugs. The latter he said would be unlawful, the former lawful.

A number of serious criticisms can be made of this reasoning. The first concerns the distinction drawn by the judge between allowing the child to die, allowing nature to take its course, and doing some positive act to bring about its death. This distinction between omissions and commissions has, of course, a respectable pedigree in the criminal law as well as providing a full and fascinating life for generations of moral philosophers. But here it is not a good distinction for two reasons. The first is that in law and in ethics, the doctor stands in a special relationship with his patient. Once he has embarked on a course of treatment, once the child is in his care, he has a duty to act affirmatively in the interests of his patient. He breaks that duty if he stands by and does nothing in circumstances in which law and ethics indicate he ought to act. Secondly, it may well be possible to argue that certain conduct amounts to an omission, but this in no way determines whether it is justified. It seeks by the use of linguistic or metaphysical sleight-of-hand to avoid the central issue: what ought the doctor to do, what is his duty?

The court could have arrived at precisely the conclusion it reached by concentrating on the notion of duty and avoiding the unsatisfactory reference to omission and commission. The question should properly have been, what is the doctor's duty to such a child? The court could then have stipulated that in certain prescribed circumstances, the doctor is not under a duty to do anything more than sedate the child and give it 'nursing care only'. The court could have decreed that the law in such circumstances absolves the doctor from a duty to feed or give drugs against infection or whatever. Not only would this be analytically more sound, but it would also save us from a future of interminable wrangles as to whether this or that conduct was or was not properly to be regarded as an omission.

My second criticism refers to the criteria which have to be satisfied before the doctor may lawfully adopt a policy of sedation and nursing care only. The court offered only two. The first was that the child be irreversibly disabled. This cannot be satisfactory. Given the consequences of the decision, it cannot be denied that such a criterion must be much more carefully defined. We must build on the court's decision so as to articulate what disabilities if any we think should qualify. Is it, for example, necessary that the child be mentally handicapped? A Down's Syndrome baby will be, but what of a spina bifida baby who may be severely physically disabled but whose mental capacities cannot be measured for weeks or months or longer, and who may turn out to be as bright as a button. Would such a baby qualify for nursing care only? Equally, irreversible disability says nothing about the severity of the disability. Is a Down's Syndrome baby with all its handicaps sufficiently seriously disabled to qualify?

The second criterion, that the parents reject the child, seems to me to be most unsatisfactory. The fate of a child, the life of a child, should not in my view depend on whether its parents want it. As *The Times*'s editorial of 6 November 1981 put it, 'Parents' wishes in these tragic circumstances deserve every respect, but they must be set against the proposition that their child is not wholly at their disposal: every live-born baby enters civil society and by doing so acquires independent rights, of which the chief concerns life itself.' The previous decision, *Re B*, in August 1981, had already made this point. That case, you will recall, concerned a baby born with Down's Syndrome who at birth also had an intestinal blockage. Surgery was needed as a matter of urgency if the child was to survive. The parents decided not to give their consent for surgery. On an application to the court by the local authority's social welfare service, the parents' decision was upheld by Mr Justice Ewbank. It was reversed by the Court of Appeal, who authorized surgery, which was then carried out. As *The Times* of 10 August argued, 'the attitude of the parents, though clearly important as a clue to the baby's prospects of affection in life, cannot be a decisive factor against treatment ... .'

It has never been part of our law or morality that parents may choose death for their children. Indeed, such a decision in other circumstances would render the parents liable to criminal prosecution and cause the child to be taken into care. This is not to ignore or belittle the enormity of the tragedy suffered by the parents. As a society we offer parents little or no support, whether in the form of practical help or professional advice, which may persuade them to keep the baby at home despite any initial decision not to do so. And the fate which awaits the baby, if it is not kept at home, is for the most part one which many parents and others would think was not far removed from a living death, lost in the back wards of some soulless institution. But this need not be, as other countries, such as Sweden, have demonstrated. In my view, to mark the child for death is to bury the problem rather than to demand we do better in terms of the care we provide, whether home support or institutional care.

My third criticism of the judge's instructions concerns his treatment of medical ethics. As we have seen, the duty a doctor owes to his patient is as much an ethical issue as a legal one. Thus it was important for the court to consider what were the relevant principles of medical ethics and to attempt to take account of these in shaping the law. But the whole of the evidence as to what good medical ethics called for in responding to a Down's Syndrome baby came from doctors, and furthermore from doctors who spoke in Dr Arthur's defence. I refer again to *The Times*'s editorial of 6 November: 'Considered as a test case in medical ethics the proceedings were not entirely satisfactory. All who offered evidence on the ethical question were broadly of one mind. Their evidence was not weighed against the views of paediatricians [and, I would interject, commentators who are not doctors] who are not of that mind, some of whom joined in the public controversy that broke out over another Down's Syndrome case which reached the Court of Appeal earlier this year' (the case of *Re B*).

The evidence offered was that it was ethically sound and acceptable to do what Dr Arthur did. No other views were heard. This omission takes on increased significance if you consult the results of the poll conducted by the BBC Television *Panorama* team. They sent out 600 questionnaires to British Consultant Paediatricians and Paediatric Surgeons. By 7 November 1981 they had received 340 replies, of which 280 were fully completed. One of the questions was: 'A Down's Syndrome baby, otherwise healthy, requires only normal care to survive: would you give it such care?' Two columns were provided for responses: one for the assumption that the parents wanted the child, the other should the parents reject the child. Ninety per cent of doctors responding on the basis of this second assumption, rejection by the parents, which is what happened in the case, said that they would give normal care. Those who said they would not do so were invited to choose between four options: a) to feed and care for it but not give it active medical treatment if it contracted a potentially fatal illness, b) to give it drugs so that it was unlikely to demand food and would eventually die, c) to give it a quick and painless death, d) don't know. *All* of the respondents, 8 per cent of the total (allowing for don't knows), opted for a). None opted for b).

Recall if you will the facts of the Arthur case. The baby was an uncomplicated Down's Syndrome baby. Evidence appeared after post-mortem that there was some damage to the child's heart, lungs and brain, but there is no evidence that this was known at the time Dr Arthur made his decision, nor is it clear that the extent of the damage was necessarily incompatible with the baby's survival, all things being equal. Dr Arthur chose sedation and nursing care only, option b) of those listed above. Not one of the doctors in the poll, which drew virtually a 50 per cent response from 600 senior paediatricians, said he would have done what Dr Arthur did, although I concede that, for obvious reasons, this is an area in which there is not always complete frankness. So it would seem that even if doctors were the arbiters of medical ethics, which I am profoundly convinced they are not, none of them in the sample regards what was done by Dr Arthur as appropriate. Nonetheless, evidence was given, and not contradicted, that it was good medical practice and good medical ethics.

Now, I come to a fourth criticism, which is of supreme importance. I shall return to it later, but it may help to take note of it here. The case seems to suggest to some, and they have greeted it as showing, that ethical dilemmas of the sort we are considering are best regarded as private matters between doctor and parent. It is said that the case lends support to the proposition that rules, principles or guidelines, call them what you will, cannot be worked out except in the vaguest, most general way. The situation is too complicated, the argument goes. The doctor and parent must be allowed to judge what to do in the light of the situation or according to the dictates of common sense. The former approach is sometimes called situation ethics; the situation dictates the response. But situations do not dictate responses, people do. The reality is that the person making the decision is bringing certain values and principles to bear, but is either unwilling or unable to articulate them. If he does so he will have to deal with the tiresome problems of resolving conflicts between clashing principles and of dealing rationally with argument and counter-argument. Equally, appeals to common sense are only valid if there is demonstrably a *common* sense, and in many of these ethical dilemmas of medicine there is decidedly no common sense. Whether or not it is realized or admitted, principles and values are being employed already in decision-making. It was the court's job to examine these and approve them, or substitute, where necessary, its own rules. It did not do this very well, but there can be no doubt that some rules do have to be laid down and followed. It is a matter of continuing astonishment to me that doctors resist the notion that there can be rules or guidelines stipulating how they ought to act. For, again whether or not it is realized or admitted, doctors are already invoking them when reaching their decisions. They do not decide in some ethical or legal vacuum. Yet still doctors resist and receive encouragement in holding what is a thoroughly untenable position. President of the Royal College of Physicians, [who] in evidence put the dilemma like this. The doctor is faced with three variables: the clinical situation of the child, which may range from normal to there being no possibility of intellectual life; the parents' attitude, which mây range from loving acceptance to revulsion; and medical management, which may range from no intervention to advanced surgery. For situations governed by three such variables *no predetermined rule and no formula of quantification was any use*' (my emphasis). I reject this emphatically.

Consider if you will the following. A policeman has the power to arrest. In exercising that power he is confronted by a number of variables. The first may be the weather and the time of day − it may

96

be foggy, snowing, icy (he should be careful if running), night, day and so on. The second variable relates to the person whom he is planning to arrest. He could be a man with a cleaver standing a few feet away, someone with a gun running towards the policeman, or an old lady in a quiet street who is clearly the worse for wear after drinking too much alcohol, and could well fall over if touched on the shoulder. A third variable could relate to the circumstances of the arrest. The person to be arrested could be at the head of a mob threatening a riot, on a picket line, or an elderly man on his own on a lonely Dorset road. A final variable may be the experience of the policeman, who may have been on the job two weeks, two months, two years or twenty years.

Does this great range of variables persuade us that we cannot establish in advance guidelines which lay down the power of arrest and reflect our ethical commitment to the freedom of the individual? Do we argue that no predetermined rule is of any use? No. We have not only drawn up ethical guidelines, we have gone further and made laws (case law and statute) setting down carefully and precisely the boundaries of permitted action allowed to the policeman who would arrest someone. The police grumble sometimes, not surprisingly. But we think it of sufficient importance to hold the balance between the supposed needs of the executive and the claims of the individual to tell the policeman that he must accept it. Certainly we would run a mile from any proposition such as, 'a policeman may arrest someone whenever he thinks it appropriate'. If a decision which affects the freedom of movement of the individual is thought so important as to warrant such attention, *a fortiori* any decision which affects not freedom of movement but life or death must attract the most careful regulation. On such analysis the argument that you cannot regulate the decision of the doctor becomes, in part at least, so much humbug.

A final criticism of the case is that it appears to leave the law in something of a mess. If my view is accepted that the law has been reshaped, it becomes necessary to reconcile it with the law propounded in the case of *Re B*. The baby in that case was more severely disabled than the boy in Dr Arthur's case, since, besides being a Down's Syndrome child, she had duodenal atresia and needed life-saving surgery. The parents had indicated that they did not want her to live and the doctors had decided not to operate. The guidance of the courts was sought and the Court of Appeal authorized the necessary surgery. As *The Times* of 10 August 1981 put it, 'It must almost inevitably be right for the court to come down on the side of life . . . ' Lord Justice Templeman decided that, 'It was wrong that the child's life should be terminated because in addition to being a mongol she had another disability.'

It appears that there is a conflict of principle here and a curious one, since the Court of Appeal's decision came first and ought ordinarily to be followed by a lower court. The cases can, I think, be reconciled, at least in principle. At one point in his judgement in *Re B*, Lord Justice Templeman put the rhetorical question, 'Is it in the best interest of the child that she should be allowed to die, or that the operation should be performed? That is the question for the court. Is the child's life going to be so demonstrably awful that it should be condemned to die; or is the kind of life so imponderable that it would be wrong to condemn her to die?' Lord Justice Templeman, on one reading of these words, is saying that, in the case before him, of a child with Down's Syndrome and an intestinal blockage, the child's life was not 'so demonstrably awful' that surgery should not be authorized. It could follow that cases could arise in which it would be right in law and medical ethics to let the child die. He did not specify in any detail what those cases may be. It could be said that in Dr Arthur's case the judge based his instructions on these words. The difficulty is, of course, that it is hard to see how they could apply to the baby in Dr Arthur's case since he was less disabled than the baby in *Re B*. Thus, a new principle may have emerged, and been correctly interpreted in Dr Arthur's case, but wrongly applied on the facts.

If we leave aside the particular facts, can we build on this new principle which has emerged from these two cases? Can we develop it into a clearer rule or set of rules for doctors to follow? This is the heart of the matter and the challenge for us. We clearly have to do better than leave decisions to be made on criteria as vague as 'irretrievably disabled' or a 'demonstrably awful' life. We first have to decide what it is about the life of a baby which would persuade us that it was ethically more justifiable to let it die than help it to live. To many, this critical criterion would be the capacity to flourish as a human being. Given the amazing number of ways which humanity finds to express itself, despite apparently crushing difficulties, I would have thought that unless there is very strong evidence, the vote must ordinarily go to life. We must ensure that the class of those marked for death is kept as narrowly and strictly defined as possible. Perhaps the key lies in the capacity to interact with others, to communicate whether rationally through language or spiritually through displays of feeling and emotion. If this criterion is accepted, and I offer it here for consideration, then we can ask a second question. How do we establish, as a matter of fact, the necessary prognosis? This is a matter of medical expertise. If, for example, we learn that a child will be able to communicate and interact but will never be free of suffering, whether physical or mental, this may cause us to consider modifying our general criterion. We may in the end decide not to, recognizing that suffering in others is hard to assess or predict and can so easily serve as a reason for choosing death for a child rather than as a challenge to our capacity to love and care. Whatever we choose, the doctor's enquiry would then be a legitimate one. He would be seeking to establish something in accordance with principles we have generally agreed upon.

This is what I see as the force of the cases of *Re B* and Dr Arthur. There are those who argue strongly, and sometimes stridently, that life is sacred, meaning by this that a child should be cared for and helped to live whatever its disability. To do otherwise, they argue, is to begin to lose respect for the lives of others and, in particular, of the disabled, whom we will more and more push into the shadows of our society. I respect this point of view but I do not share it. And, unhappily, it is unlikely that we shall ever arrive at a consensus here, just as in a number of other troubling medical ethical issues, such as abortion. Where this is so, we may, indeed must, choose a position which is rationally defensible, not offensive to the majority, and which will work in practice. A respectable ethical argument can, I submit, be made out for not striving to keep alive those babies who soon after birth can be shown to have no capacity ever to flourish as human beings. Modern medicine has brought us to the point where almost all babies are salvageable in some form. But simply because we can do so, does not mean we must. We have never as a society regarded the preservation of life as an absolute value in itself. We admit the notion of the just war, and we praise, rather than condemn, the hero who sacrifices his life in a good cause. We also concede that no one has an absolute right to life, since the just war may warrant its being taken, as may capital punishment or the action of a ship's captain in closing bulkheads to save his ship and its passengers, even though some crew on the wrong side of the bulkhead will drown. On the other hand, we do not think that life should be taken lightly. It is something of fundamental value to us. Thus, it should only be taken, or someone should only be left to die, if a very good reason exists. If you apply this reasoning to the newborn you will see that, while he has no absolute right to life, he should be helped to live unless there is a very good reason not to do so. A demonstrable incapacity to flourish as a human being in the sense in which I have sketched it out earlier, would in my view amount to such a reason.

Once articulated, these ethical rules would equally apply to other situations in which the quality of life is an issue. For example, in the case of the terminally ill, they would offer a guide to the doctor as to whether he is ethically and legally obliged to intervene if pneumonia or cardiac arrest strikes the patient with advanced cancer. If the patient is otherwise unconscious or so drugged, out of necessity, as to be out of contact with the world, or is racked by pain, it could be said that his capacity to flourish as a human being is lost. This would provide the justification for letting nature take its course.

What if someone not yet *in extremis* decides of his own volition that he wishes to die now rather than await the degrading decline he fears? Do the principles we have begun to map out apply to him, such that if he is asked, his doctor may help him to achieve his death? The case of *R* v. *Reed* serves as a caution. The British Euthanasia Society, Exit, is a society which exists to disseminate information to any member of the Society on how to take his life. In October 1981, the Secretary of the Society was convicted of the crime of aiding and abetting the suicide of several people, all of whom had contacted the Society, as they were contemplating suicide, but were fearful that they might make a mess of things. He was sentenced to two and a half years in prison. Undoubtedly he broke the law. There was, however, no effort on the part of the judge to reshape the law, or so interpret it as to avoid conviction. Further, the sentence was intended as a warning to others. I invite you to stand back and consider what this prosecution and conviction says about our society when contrasted with the case of Dr Arthur. Elderly and, in some cases, ill people formed an intention to kill themselves. They made an autonomous choice — perhaps, for them, the final act of self-determination. They feared more than anything ending their days in a hospital bed, shorn of any dignity, prevented from dying, the reluctant recipients of all that modern medicine can deliver. There can be no doubt that this is a very real fear for many, whether it is justified or not. So they sought advice and were given it. They chose to die. And their helper was sent to jail.

Would it have made any difference if their helper had been a doctor? As a matter of legal principle, it would not. The aiding and abetting of suicide would still be a crime. But in practice it would have made all the difference in the world. First, there would not have been the fanfare of publicity which surrounded Exit's activities, promoted in part by Exit. Instead, there would have been a discussion between doctor and patient. Secondly, the means chosen for the comfortable death would have been different: more subtle and carefully managed. Thirdly, the doctor would have undoubtedly been able to call on medical experts who could show that the dosage of drugs used was not outside the norm of treatment, or did not cause, or may not have caused, the death. And so on. I have no doubt that many doctors have responded to a request for assistance and helped a patient to ease his way towards death. I am not criticizing them. I believe it can be defended as a humane and caring act in certain carefully limited circumstances. What is important here is to notice the ethical and legal implications of the Exit case. Surely it cannot be explained simply on the basis that in the Exit case there was no doctor. For doctors, as we have seen, enjoy no special privileges. But when a doctor stands by and allows a baby to die, because the child is disabled and unwanted, professionals are tumbling over themselves to defend him and to praise him (at least in public) and he is acquitted. There was no question of any autonomous decision by the baby. He had no part in the proceedings. If we excuse those who choose death for babies, who cannot speak for themselves, we should be slow to punish those who facilitate the autonomous decision of someone to destroy himself. Alternatively, we must live with the charge of hypocrisy, or even one law for the professional and one for the rest.

I make no apologies for dwelling on this particular problem for so long. Not only is it intrinsically important, but it is also necessary to try to tease out the direction law and ethics may be taking. But I want to end the discussion as I began, and remind you of the theme we started with. I can do no better than adopt the words of Mr Justice Kirby, the outstanding Chairman of the Australian Law Reform Commission. In an address to the Royal Australasian College of Physicians in November 1981 he said, 'If we are to sanction procedures by which, in certain cases, grossly deformed or profoundly retarded children are not to be given the medical facilities which would be routine and unquestioned in a normal child, we may, in practical terms, be deciding that the deformed and retarded will die.

That may be the right decision. The community which has to contribute significantly to the support of such a child may have its own legitimate moral claim to be heard on the subject. But, as it seems to me, these decisions should not be left to the unarticulated judgement of individual medical practitioners. They should not be left to secret in-house rules designed by hospitals or their ethics committees and varying among them. They should not be left to the undefined collective of the Medical Profession, still less should they respond to strident appeals for confidence in medical professionalism. Decisions of life and death, even of a retarded or disabled child, even of an old person on the brink of death, are too important to be abandoned in this way.'

Compare, if you will, the words of Dr John Havard, secretary of the British Medical Association. On 21 October 1981, he delivered a speech at the BMA's annual conference, which he called 'Legal threats to Medicine'. It was given in that section of the conference entitled 'Medicine in Jeopardy'. In his somewhat intemperate and casually argued address, which had all the qualities of a rallying call to the besieged faithful, Dr Havard spoke of doctors being 'hounded' by the courts of law, though no evidence of this was offered. He was anxious to alert his members to the 'threat which law presents to modern medical practice.' His conclusion echoes views we have already noticed and will hear of again later. 'It should be a matter of considerable concern,' he said, 'to the medical profession that the courts are attempting, and attempting with considerable success, to influence clinical and ethical decisions, bearing in mind that these decisions have to be taken by doctors at a time when they have no way of knowing for certain what the outcome will be.' Little, if anything, is known for certain. We all work on best estimates. And we develop guidelines for conduct on the basis of those estimates.

Now let me turn to another ethical issue. Let me remind you of what I said earlier: that you would not ordinarily accept it as proper that doctors alone should decide when principles of honesty should be observed or waived.

Consider Mrs X. She has cancer. It is decided that the cancer will not respond to treatment and that she will die within a matter of weeks or months. Given that such predictions are at best guesses, the question that then arises in the mind of her doctor is what he should tell her. Should he tell her the truth about her condition, or offer some alternative story which is perhaps more optimistic? I choose the example of cancer, as it is familiar. Of course, the questions raised are by no means limited to cancer patients. They pervade the whole range of medical care. The Royal Commission on the NHS makes the point that 31 per cent of in-patients and 25 per cent of out-patients in a specially commissioned survey did not consider they were given enough information about their treatment and care.

The assumptions which underlie these questions about what to tell Mrs X, are obvious. People do not want to die; neither do they want to know they are dying; nor could they tolerate being told they are dying; nor do they know they are dying. Some or even all of these assumptions may be well founded on occasion, but they are unsupported by any evidence. They reflect the anxieties of the healthy. As Susan Sontag writes in her book *Illness as Metaphor*, 'All this lying to cancer patients is a measure of how much harder it has become in advanced industrial societies to come to terms with death.' In fact, as Una MacLean points out in her paper, 'Learning about Death', in the *Journal of Medical Ethics* of June 1980, what surveys there are, show that the large majority of patients with, for example, cancer would prefer to know the truth. By contrast, doctors, she found, ordinarily choose not to tell, preferring silence, half-truths, or even, occasionally, untruths.

Perhaps the most important assumption underlying the question of what to tell the patient is that it is the doctor who is uniquely qualified to decide what the patient should know. Of course, once the view is allowed that patients do not want to know the truth, rationalizations can readily be created which serve to justify this position. The notion that the patient does not wish to know soon becomes the notion that the patient should not know. One argument commonly used is that the diagnosis is uncertain. But a study by J. McIntosh published in 1978 by the Institute of Medical Sociology in Aberdeen, in the book *Relationships between Doctors and Patients*, demonstrated that uncertainty over diagnosis was not the reason for withholding information, though it was used to justify it. The better explanation for non-communication, according to McIntosh, was uncertainty, not over diagnosis, but over how much each patient wished to know, an uncertainty largely produced by the doctor's own anxieties. All the doctors in the study firmly believed that the great majority of patients should not be told that they had cancer, nor be given their prognosis unless it was favourable. The patients were to be given only as much information as was compatible with the retention of hope, whether justified or not. The doctors realized that some patients may indeed have wished to know the truth, but, since without asking they could not know which patients, they managed the problem by not telling anyone, unless a patient specifically demanded the truth. This may have provided the ideal coping mechanism for the doctors. But it meant that only the patient who was articulate, who insisted on the truth, and was confident enough to be persistent, got his way.

Another rationalization resorted to is the so-called therapeutic privilege. This suggests that, as a matter of good medical practice, the doctor may withhold information from the patient if, in the exercise of his discretion and judgement, it would not be in the best interests of the patient's health to know. This is clearly a device created by doctors to do what is in the best interests of doctors. It may be justified on some occasions, but there is no effort to specify these occasions. Everything proceeds on the basis of the particular doctor's judgement. It all boils down to the doctor being good, gentle and kind. It would be nice if all our doctors were like this. But, just in case, can we not have some more certain guarantees that our interests, as defined by us, may be allowed to prevail? The device of the therapeutic privilege pays lip service to the principles of truth-telling and self-determination, while it creates a discretionary exception which is quite capable of swallowing these principles when the doctor decides the occasion requires it.

If we look beneath these rationalizations we see a principle being observed which is certainly not part of received tradition concerning the doctor–patient relationship. The traditional view is that the doctor–patient relationship rests on trust, or at least on agreement. But what we see is an operational principle, defined by the doctor and accepted by us by default, which allows the doctor to suspend the trust, or rewrite the agreement, when in his view this is appropriate. Of course, if the patient breaks his trust or violates the agreement there may be dire consequences for him, even to the extent of forfeiting further care. Not so for the doctor. He remains arbiter of the relationship, even to the extent of claiming the privilege of resorting to an operational principle which is the precise opposite of traditional ethics. For it is a basic moral principle of our society that we should tell the truth. If this principle is to be the subject of exceptions, and it is, of course, well recognized that there are circumstances in which it is justified to withhold the truth, or even to lie, this should only be after careful analysis and common agreement. No one is saying it is easy to tell the truth. It is a difficult, even harrowing task. It has to be managed with great sensitivity. It calls for the exercise of considerable skill and understanding. This is part of the doctor's job. This is what he should be trained to do, rather than follow the lead of those who urge that the truth may be nudged and fudged. Yet he rarely receives anything but the most rudimentary training. The consequence is that, despite their central importance, the doctor very often has a less than adequate command of communication skills, as Professor Fletcher has shown in his book, *Talking with Patients*. So, fudging and nudging the truth go on and are defended.

Only recently, in the *Journal of Medical Ethics* of June 1982, two doctors involved in clinical trials of drugs offered various defences for not telling patients that they were the subjects of research. Dr Raanon Gillon, the learned editor of the Journal, in his excellent editorial, reminded us that, if we accept the view that doctors should not lie to or deliberately deceive their patients, then the view that 'misinformed' consent' can be sanctioned 'is untenable'. Only two months previously, *The Times* of 22 April 1982 carried a story of the death of an 85-year-old woman who had been involved, without her knowledge, in a trial for the treatment of cancer. It had been decided not to tell her after consultation between the doctors involved and their local ethics committees. Dr Michael Thomas, Chairman of the Central Ethical Committee of the British Medical Association, was reported as saying that 'there are occasions when seeking consent might prejudice the trial'. 'The trials', he went on, showed the 'possibility of a major breakthrough in the treatment of cancer.' Dr Gillon comments on this argument in his editorial. 'Of course', he wrote, 'it does not follow that the research should therefore go ahead *without* obtaining informed consent.' The issue to him is, 'whether or not the doctor in such circumstances intends to put that particular patient's interests above all other considerations'.

The principle of truth-telling is part of our ethical tradition not only because it is the only basis on which trust can be based. Once someone is deceived, and discovers the deceit, the possibility for trust is destroyed. We cling to it because it also enables a person to have autonomy, to have control over his life. We respect his need for autonomy because we assume that he is ordinarily the best judge of his own interests. If he knows the truth, he is then best placed to respond according to what he sees as his best interests. To deny him information is to deny him autonomy. It is to rob him of his power to act as he thinks best. It enables the doctor to act as he, the doctor, thinks best. Thus, it is the doctor's ethical duty to tell his patient the truth. Only in exceptional circumstances may it be withheld. One such circumstance would be when the patient has unequivocally indicated that he does not want to know, that he has waived his right to autonomy. As Dr Gillon put it in his editorial, the common view is that 'doctors must *not* lie to or deliberately deceive their patients, even though they should be sensitive about not thrusting *unwanted* truths at patients'. Other exceptions may exist. Clearly, they must be the product of careful analysis. They cannot rest on the unexamined and unarticulated say-so of the doctor.

The examples I have referred to so far are fairly commonplace. We would all have recognized them as typical of medical practice, even if we may not all have recognized the ethical nature of the decisions made. It may be that some of you would still be content to leave things as they are, despite the far-reaching significance of such decisions. Well, let me press you a little further. Let me press the point that decisions taken by doctors are of such a nature that a check should exist on the power this decision-making grants to them. I want now to look not at specific examples but across a whole area of medical practice — that concerned with reproduction and birth. I want to identify for you the ethical principles by reference to which this area of medicine is practised. You may not as easily recognize the decisions which are made as being part of traditional doctoring. They seem far more clearly for us to make, rather than leave to the doctor alone. Perhaps, when you have heard what I suggest, you will be more prepared to accept my thesis, that doctors are involved in making decisions which are more than technical. They are ethical decisions about us. They closely affect our lives. They are made without reference to agreed principles. They invest great power in the doctor. And they are regarded, at least by doctors, as uniquely within their competence to make, such that their power is not easily checked.

So let us turn to medical practice concerned with reproduction and birth. Let me quickly suggest some of the contexts in which medicine is involved, and in which decisions are made by doctors. Obviously there is abortion. Then there is the treatment of severely handicapped newly-born babies which I have already mentioned. Then there is the screening of pregnant mothers and foetuses to identify deviations from the chosen norm. There is the provision of genetic counselling to parents, to help those who may bear a disabled child to make their decision whether or not to have a child. There is medicine aimed at inducing fertility, for example artificial insemination and, most recently, *in vitro* fertilization, the so-called test-tube baby. And there is contraception which includes, of course, sterilization. On careful analysis, decisions taken by doctors in these areas of medicine, despite the superficial differences, can be shown to rest upon certain underlying common assumptions which are ethical in nature. I suggest, furthermore, that these common ethical assumptions are unstated, unarticulated and certainly unremarked, because it is probably not appreciated by doctors or others that they are being made. Yet, when they are identified, they can be shown to be of very great significance, reflecting and affecting as they do our approach to child-bearing and the value of life. You may well wish to reflect upon who it is who should decide whether you are fit to raise children.

Consider what Professor Henry Miller wrote in his book *Medicine and Society*; that final decisions on such matters as planned parenthood rest often with parents, but, 'the trouble is, of course, that the parents from whom difficult decisions are most likely to be required are all too often drawn from the most feckless and irresponsible sections of the population'. 'The problematical issue of positive as opposed to negative eugenic policy', he goes on, ' . . . is fatally complicated by the fact that, unlike the breeders of horses for courses, we don't and can't really know exactly what we want: the qualities desirable in a 1918 infantryman are not necessarily those appropriate to an astronaut.' You are left in little doubt as to what should happen if we did or could know what qualities were needed!

The first common, underlying assumption is that some are more fit than others for child-bearing and child-raising, with the implication that the unfit should not bear or raise children. But, if we were to attempt abstractly to devise a set of criteria of fitness to be a parent, I doubt if we would get very far. Clearly what is at the heart of the assumption is a concern for the potential child. A child just should not be born into a particular environment or to particular parents. Yet there is an extraordinary ambivalence in how this concern is demonstrated. On the one hand, it seems to be reflected in a doctor's decision to sterilize the mentally retarded girl before she can get pregnant and bear a child whose future may be less than happy. And the decision by doctors to offer artificial insemination only to stable married couples who have passed some sort of parental fitness test seems to express the same concern for the welfare of future children. Equally, Steptoe and

Edwards, developers of the latest reproductive technology of *in vitro* fertilization, have announced that they have drawn up a code of practice whereby, according to *The Times* of 14 July 1980, potential beneficiaries will have to pass the same sort of parental fitness test. Parenthood is to be encouraged, indeed facilitated, but only in certain circumstances. It is to be prevented in others. The guiding criterion is concern for future children.

But the ambivalence creeps in when a doctor with these views refuses a woman's request for an abortion, just as much a medical practice in the area of reproduction as are the others. Where is the concern for the future child there? Or where is it when he refuses to prescribe contraceptive pills to a girl who is under sixteen? The doctor doubtless regards her as unfit to be a mother, to bring a child into the world, but his decision not to prescribe the contraceptive pills may well have precisely this effect.

In these last two cases, the ethical principles of fitness to be a parent and concern for the fate of the child, which previously guided the doctor, seem lost, though arguably these are situations in which application of them would be more than appropriate. Instead he seems to be operating on another ethical principle, that a woman ought to bear the child conceived. Whether it is in the child's best interest to be born is suddenly of less importance. It is almost as if the birth of the child is seen as punishment, that it is no more than is deserved. There is, in effect, a complicated intermingling of a whole set of principles or, some would say, prejudices or biases. On the one hand, there is a policy of eugenics, seeking the right parents. But, on the other hand, there is a policy of retribution, whereby children must be brought into the world regardless. And these policies are completely within the power of doctors to operate.

As Lesley Doyal points out in her book *The Political Economy of Health*, it is clear that in the case, for example, of abortion doctors operate a system of screening of women which has nothing at all to do with the legal requirements for abortion laid down in the Abortion Act 1967. Single women seem to be divided into 'the girl who made a mistake' and 'the bad girl'. Women have to be very careful in their management of their relationship with their doctor. If the good girl is suitably contrite she gets her abortion. The bad girl does not. It would only encourage her to be promiscuous. Doyal quotes the remarkable conclusions of a study of Scottish doctors:

'Not unnaturally, the doctor does not like it if he and the help he can give seem to be taken for granted. The wording of her request, the wrong manner, too demanding or over-confident, even her way of walking in ("she comes prancing in") may antagonize him and lessen her chances of referral. On the other hand, too passive an approach can be misinterpreted. "You get the impression with a lot of these lassies that you could push them one way or the other and in a situation like this I tend to say keep the baby . . . " The doctors respond best to a concerned approach and tears are never amiss.'

The ethics involved are crude and contradictory. Yet they pass, unstated and unchallenged, as part of the practice of reproductive medicine. We happily leave it all to the doctors and should not be surprised at the idiosyncratic and contradictory principles which emerge.

A second ethical assumption which underlies medical thinking and practice concerned with reproduction and birth is that a baby should not be born or, if born, should not be encouraged to live, if the quality of life the child would enjoy falls below a certain standard. Of course, the first observation is that what amounts to a minimum quality of life is not adequately analysed, far less authoritatively set out. And, as we have seen, there is no lack of resistance to such attempts to lay down rules and guidelines. I have already explored the point and offered some views. But the debate has really only just begun, at the level of thoughtful and public comment. Yet I am suggesting that this principle, inarticulate and idiosyncratic as it may still be, is one of the most significant guiding principles in this area of medical practice. Once again, the alleged motive is concern for the child. We can see this clearly in the practice of selective treatment of severely handicapped newly-born babies. The most severely handicapped do not receive surgery or antibiotics and are encouraged to die peacefully, or, to use the words of Dr John Lorber, one of the most famous specialists, the babies are not encouraged to live. This same concern for the child is also reflected in the law and practice of abortion, where there is less than the usual opposition when abortion on the grounds that the child will be genetically severely handicapped is raised. Furthermore, the modern practice of screening pregnant mothers is posited on this assumption, that it would not be in the interests of the child if it were born genetically disabled.

In tandem with the enormous development of the field of genetics in the past two decades we have also witnessed the appearance of genetic counselling. There cannot be much doubt that here too, this same assumption operates. Of course, the theory is that the mother should be given the information and then left to make up her own mind. The role of the doctor involved is allegedly that of a neutral purveyor of facts, rather than an advocate of any particular decision. I doubt if this distinction is real, since no presentation of facts is value-free, and the so-called neutral party can always, by the facts he chooses to relay and the emphasis he places upon them, manipulate effectively the decision arrived at.

Few would suggest that this ethical assumption concerning a minimum quality of life is wholly wrong or ought to be abandoned. But, quite apart from its present clear lack of definition, it is important to notice the eugenic tone which underlies it. There is, perhaps, some moral danger in following a path which leads to the conclusion that the handicapped should not be born. Though we all want healthy children, health, as we know, is a term which defies easy definition. And who is to say at what point of the scale of handicap a baby's life would not be worth living in the absence of evidence, since the child is in the womb, of the capacity to develop mentally? Furthermore, such a pursuit of the handicap-free child might inevitably make us less tolerant of that child who, for whatever reason, is not caught by the screening process. Is such a child to face a future as a freak or a reject, shunned, because such children are just not born like that any more?

And there is again some ambivalence in medical attitude and practice in this context. Those doctors who refuse to perform an abortion to prevent the birth of a genetically disabled child also claim that they are concerned only with the child's best interests. But, to them, there is no minimum quality to a child's life. Only in such a way, they seem to argue, can we remain a caring society, rather than a selfish and narcissistic one which only wants babies if they are made in the right image. Existence is all — a view shared by those doctors who advocate that severely handicapped newly-born babies should be helped to live, rather than encouraged to die. But even these doctors might perform an abortion for a girl who had been horribly raped, or draw the line at treating the most severely handicapped newly-born baby. So, while differing from other doctors, their own position also is not free from ambivalence.

These issues concerning a minimum quality of life are profoundly difficult. What is striking is that, despite their significance, they are not widely discussed. They are resolved in the consulting-room and debated, if at all, in the medical journals. But, as you have seen, the ethical assumption that there is a certain minimum quality of life is unclear. The counter-principle, that there is no minimum quality of life, co-exists with it, again with no clear meaning or clue as to when one, rather than the other, should operate, producing ambivalence and contradiction. What adds to these problems is that in this, as in so many other areas of medicine, science and technology have developed their own momentum. New procedures such as foetal screening are introduced because they are now possible. Any consideration of the ethical implications is seen as quite independent and usually, if undertaken, takes the form of capitulation before another technological *fait accompli*.

A third underlying ethical assumption, I suggest, is that a child has a certain worth, socially and economically, and should be conceived, or born, only if it would qualify as worth it. This is most evident in the case of abortion, when a doctor may find himself asked to certify that the birth of a child would be a detriment to the existing family's health. Here, the word 'health' can be manipulated, if need be, to include the threat to the health of existing children represented by additional competition for the available resources of the family. Here the underlying concern may be, as in other cases, for the child about to be born; that he is better off not born. But there seems to be an equal concern for those children already born. Those who oppose abortion are particularly concerned at the extent to which this criterion is capable of being manipulated. It means that the decision whether a child should be born may be made to depend on the social convenience of the birth. But to argue otherwise is to say that the child should be born, even though it would not be welcome.

Despite the complexity of the argument and the conflict of principles, we can once again find doctors making decisions, giving advice, as if what was involved was a mere matter of technical expertise. Any ethical analysis which is indulged in is rudimentary at best and not exposed to wider scrutiny. Indeed, recently, doctors specializing in the field of reproduction have found themselves more and more parleyed into these ethical difficulties. Through the development of foetal screening, they have been able to discover more and more about the foetus, so as to aid the parents in deciding what course to take. Now comes the problem. What if a doctor knows that Mr and Mrs X want desperately to have a baby boy? In the course of routine screening, he discovers that the foetus Mrs X is carrying is healthy, but a female. Doctors have got themselves into a considerable lather about whether or not the parents should be told this when it is likely, in our chosen hypothesis, that the mother will then seek to have the foetus aborted. The doctor may not regard the information as relevant to any decision the parents may wish to make. But, by defining what is relevant, the doctor is already making a judgement that only certain information should be revealed and that he should be the sole judge of this. To lie, to withhold the information, or to reveal it — each is equally repugnant to many doctors. This is, if you will, another example of the dilemmas medical technology brings in its wake. We must, it is clear, flush out these ethical problems associated with medicine at the beginning of life. They affect our future, they are ours to resolve.

So let me tie up the various threads of my argument. We have seen how decisions made by doctors are ethical in nature, calling for careful analysis. There is little evidence that such analysis is engaged in. If, for instance, you look for wise words and advice to the recently revised *Handbook of Medical Ethics* produced by the British Medical Association, you will be disappointed. For example, the section on the treatment of severely handicapped children ends in the ringing phrase, 'the doctor must find a just and humane solution for the infant and the family'. So far, so good; but just what is a just solution? To argue, as some doctors do, that 'we learn on the job' is to support some notion of education by osmosis, or to say that they perpetuate, un-considered, the views of their predecessors, or to admit that they receive no education at all in ethics.

We should expect that doctors have some educational grounding in ethical analysis. To suggest this last crucial point has been, until very recently, to invite scorn. 'There is no room in the curriculum. We do not want to clutter up our timetable with well-meaning Sunday school exercises.' My response is that much greater stress must be laid on the humanities during a doctor's training. Ethics must be a central course, taught not by some superannuated elder statesman, nor by the latest medical star in the firmament, but by an outsider, someone who is not deafened by the rhetoric of medicine. Medical schools must simply be dragged back into our world and out of their hermetically sealed cocoon of a world, in which we are counters with which the game of life is played. There is, at last, some indication that this message is being heard. Since 1980, there has been a definite quicken-ing of interest in teaching ethics to medical students and to recently qualified GPs. Much of the teaching still takes the form of the occasional guest lecture. There is still no medical school which has, as a required course, a formal, rigorous study of medical ethics. But I detect an inevitable movement in that direction, a movement for which medical students have not been slow to show their support. And I would go further. The teaching of medical ethics should also feature in postgraduate and Royal College training. It was, after all, Hippocrates who said that every physician should be a philosopher.

What I have said will be thoroughly unobjectionable, as well as self-evident, to many. But it is important to realize that hostility to the study of medical ethics remains strong. Objections are still raised to considering it in any depth. Let me note briefly some of these objections. First, ethics does not figure prominently in the education of doctors, perhaps because it is thought that there is a danger that philosophical discourse on such a subject can soon wander off into abstraction and logic-chopping, far removed from the realities of life. Certainly, many doctors are tempted to be wary of the subject, to doubt its importance, its relevance, to bracket it with art appreciation or structuralism as toys for academics to play with. I would make the point, therefore, that while we must discuss often complex issues of moral philosophy we must always deal with real life. We must discover and seek to understand the facts of medical practice and make whatever principles we develop respond to these. We must, in short, keep our feet firmly on the ground.

Another reason for hostility to the study of medical ethics lies in the role doctors see themselves and are seen by others as having; they are *doers*, they must respond to what is presented. This suggests that contemplation is an unavailable luxury, even that it is dangerous. The doctor may argue that he has no time to ponder the niceties of the concepts of autonomy or consent when a pregnant woman, who happens to be a Jehovah's Witness, is bleeding to death. And the education of doctors tends to reinforce this, dealing as it does in assertion, analysing problems through resort to check-lists. The philosopher, on the other hand, like the lawyer, is weaned on pro-position and counter-proposition, on the inevitability, even the desir-ability, of conflict and uncertainty. As a consequence of this education and self-perception, the doctor will be temperamentally disinclined to look with favour on medical ethics. This I think is unfortunate. The supposed gulf between the thinker and the doer is not real. The moral philosopher must persuade the doctor that he is there to help, to make the doctor's life easier, when it comes to making hard decisions. For if, prior to confronting situations, the doctor has been introduced to the rigours of ethical analysis and been assisted in untangling competing and conflicting claims, he will be that much more prepared to deal with the situation when it arises. He will need to agonize less. The burden he feels is put upon him to decide what to do will weigh less heavily. Take the well-known problem of the girl under 16 who seeks a prescription for contraceptive pills. Her GP, who, let us imagine, is the family doctor, may think it right to inform her parents. This is a matter of some ethical complexity. Should the GP seek the girl's consent? If she refuses, may he ignore her refusal? What is left of confidentiality if he tells the parents without asking permission of the girl? Does he, by telling the parents, breach the trust she vests in him and break his promise to keep her consultation secret? Is he justified in breaking this trust on the ground, for example, that a greater good is served by doing so than by remaining quiet? Is it right to consider the greater good, and who should be the arbiter of this? Can there be a hierarchy of values in which trust and consent and autonomy are ranked lower than enforcing and reflecting a particular view of family life, or conforming to a particular set of sexual mores? This is the stuff of medical ethics. It is hard but it can be resolved, so that the doctor may have rationally defensible options which do not do violence to moral principles. For the doctor to say that this is so much hot air, that common sense or experience tell you the answer, is, I submit, to do an injustice to the moral claims of the patient and to fall below the high standards of professionalism which the profession properly sets itself.

Jonathan Glover in his book *Causing Death and Saving Lives*, makes the point when he writes, in his delightful style, that some may say 'it is as pointless to argue about morality as it would be to try to persuade someone by argument to prefer one colour to another'. 'But', he says, 'this is to take too pessimistic a view.' He then indicates a number of ways in which moral arguments can be tested. For example, they may rest on a blurred or incoherent concept, such as the word 'unnatural'. If someone using it in an argument against homosexuality were 'pressed to define "unnatural"', he may find it hard to provide a definition that includes homosexual acts without also including singing at the opera'. Other methods Glover cites are 'the exposure of logical inadequacies', or showing someone 'that his beliefs have unnoticed consequences that he would find unacceptable', such as an argument in support of abortion which would equally justify infanticide.

If the dangers of over-abstraction or remoteness from real life are avoided, there would seem to be no *principled* reason why medical ethics should not be taken seriously. But, unfortunately, there are still those engaged in medicine who offer objections to the study of medical ethics, who reject it as not worthwhile. This rejection, since it does not rest on principle, grows, as Sisela Bok suggests in her very helpful paper, 'The tools of bioethics', out of two emotions — resentment and the sense of being threatened. While both may be understandable, it is crucial that they be overcome. The doctor, Bok argues, resents what he sees as the intrusion of outsiders and perceives it as a threat to his professional status. This is so despite the fact that we have seen that, in matters of ethics, the non-doctor is not an outsider, and that he is not interfering, but trying to help.

This resentment and sense of being threatened cause doctors to give the impression that theirs is a beleaguered profession. It is as if they were under siege from a hostile and unsympathetic world. And this, in turn, may find itself translated into a hostility or objection to the very notion that there can be rules in the context of medical ethics. The recoil of many doctors at the word rule is born of a fairly primitive territoriality and professional defensiveness. Rules prescribe what ought to or must be done. They would, in other words, many doctors reason unthinkingly, be telling us what to do. They would, and here appears the magic word, control us doctors. And control, of course, threatens professional dignity and licence and therefore must be resisted. If you think this is an overstatement I would exchange your experience with mine as I have travelled about talking and listening. A somewhat more sophisticated resistance takes the form we have already seen in Sir Douglas Black's comments in the Dr Arthur trial, that rules would be nice, but they are impossible given the variations in facts which the doctor is presented with.

Each of these positions is naive and ignores what already goes on. It is naive or, perhaps, disingenuous, in that the assumption is made that the practice of medicine is, or can be made, rule-less. A moment's reflection will be enough to persuade you that all social interaction is regulated by rules. They are not to be feared nor can they be avoided. Twining and Miers point out, in their fascinating book *How to Do Things With Rules*, that 'there is hardly any aspect of human behaviour that is not in some way governed or at least guided by rules'. Whether it is playing chess, entering a room, remonstrating with a neighbour or examining a patient, rules exist setting out the limits of tolerated conduct. They exist to serve a number of purposes. In the context of the doctor's relationship with his patient, they provide, among other things, the basis on which the consultation may be conducted. They serve as a guarantee to doctor and patient that certain standards will be observed, as a reference point from which to judge the behaviour of the doctor and the patient and as the link whereby the partnership between the two can be established. As for the proposition that the variability of facts makes rules impossible, this ignores the way social life is ordinarily organized. It is a commonplace that rules are couched in general terms and must be applied to specific facts. In this application, room is usually left for the proper exercise of discretion in keeping with the spirit of the rule. We are familiar with such rules as 'a player may be penalized for ungentlemanly conduct', or 'a barrister must not bring his profession into disrepute', or 'a doctor must exercise reasonable care'. We live with these and over time build up a knowledge of what may be ungentlemanly, disreputable, or un-reasonable. Equally, it is a commonplace that we place fact-situations into categories. This obviates the need for having a rule for each situation. For example, we can talk of emergencies, or clinical trials, or of cold surgery, or of the chronically ill, the new-born and the geriatric. Emergencies, because of their nature, may call for special rules as to how a doctor must behave, but we do not need, nor do we have, a separate ethical rule depending on whether the emergency involves a broken leg, a cardiac arrest or an epileptic fit, nor on whether the patient is Mr Jones, Mr Smith or Mr Brown. Just as they fall into categories for the purposes of deciding on treatment so they do as regards the rules which specify how, in terms of ethics, the doctor must behave. After all, did not Dr Arthur put the baby boy in his care into a category earmarked for nursing care only, because he was born with Down's Syndrome and his parents did not want him to survive?

Professor Herbert Hart puts it this way in *The Concept of Law*: 'If it were not possible to communicate general standards of conduct, which multitudes of individuals could understand, without further direction, as requiring from them certain conduct when occasion arose, nothing that we now recognize as law could exist. Hence the law must predominantly, but by no means exclusively, refer to *classes* of persons, and to *classes* of acts, things and circumstances; and its successful operation over vast areas of social life depends on a widely diffused capacity to recognize particular acts, things and circumstances as instances of the general classifications which the law (or any other system of rules) makes.' Of course, it is crucial to add that anyone claiming that the situation before him constitutes an exception to the ordinary rule, must first be able to defend this claim, and, secondly, identify the rule which governs the exception, since exceptions do not float about free of all regulation.

Having got some of these objections out of the way, you may still ask what will doctors and medical students get out of a study of medical ethics? What, if you will, is medical ethics all about? The teaching of ethics would introduce future doctors to the sort of tension and even contradiction between ethical principles which I have been trying to illustrate. The claim that there is only one fundamental professional ethic, 'benefit and above all do no harm', would be exposed as untenable. For example, a Jehovah's Witness in danger of bleeding to death may refuse a blood transfusion, fully aware of the implications of his decision. If there were only one ethical principle in the practice of medicine and if it were solely for the doctor to dictate and interpret, it could justify ignoring the patient's decision. But, in fact, we tend to favour the ethical principle of respect for an individual's autonomy and freedom, whatever the doctor or others may wish to do. And there are other ethical principles we hold in equally strong regard. One very important one is the principle of doing justice within society by, for instance, avoiding discrimination and allocating resources fairly. This is important because it suggests that the traditional notion of the doctor's duty being to his patient, and only to his patient, should not go unchallenged. For if justice includes the fair allocation of resources within the community, it may mean that the interests of a particular patient must properly be weighed against the larger interests of the community, and that, in appropriate cases, the doctor should put the community first. This, as I have said, is the stuff of medical ethics, exploring the tensions and conflicts between ethical principles and suggesting ways of resolving them. This is the sort of rigorous analysis to which medical students and doctors must be introduced.

Here is not the place to embark on any detailed examination of medical ethics. That is a task for specialist works. There is always a danger that brief sallies into the field serve only to trivialize what is a complex area. They tend to titillate the voyeur who likes to ponder the

117

problems rather than serve the doctor and the community who have to find answers. It is for this reason that I have previously avoided any attempt to offer some sort of primer or introduction to medical ethics. While I am still persuaded that this is the right course to adopt here, I would like to take a few moments to look somewhat more closely at some of the themes I mentioned just now. As I do so, please take note of the type of fact-situation we consider. Medical ethics is concerned with the everyday practice of medicine. Indeed, it could be argued that 80–90 per cent of the problems GPs have to deal with are fundamentally ethical in nature. All too often, unfortunately, medical ethics is represented as revolving around such medical exotica as heart transplants, *in vitro* fertilization or transsexualism. There are enough difficult ethical problems in day-to-day practice without referring to such exotica, which in any event make the analysis advanced seem as remote as the procedure being discussed.

I begin with a declaration of my ideal which I hope is also yours – to seek the ethical principles which will allow for the most morally defensible and successful relationship between doctor and patient. Such a relationship to my mind involves a sharing of responsibility between doctor and patient and a considered respect for principles such as autonomy, dignity, justice, the doing of good and avoiding of harm. The present basis of medical ethics is not in my view designed to achieve this end. It does not offer a sound basis for good medical ethics. It provides an inappropriate model for the relationship of doctor and patient. It is time we considered how to establish a sounder set of medical ethical principles.

Before doing so, let me recapitulate briefly what I have said so far. I have already indicated that I am satisfied that medical ethics is an area in which non-doctors, aware of the facts of medical practice and trained in appropriate disciplines, must be allowed to play their part. I have also indicated my view that education in ethics must be an essential part of medical training. Doctors need not be threatened by this nor need they resent it as interference. Instead, all will benefit – the future patient, society in general and the doctor, who at present is left to muddle through some awesomely difficult problems and often criticized whatever he does. The proper study of medical ethics will produce guidelines for future conduct, tools for analysis which will forearm the doctor. Finally, I must make it clear again that I am not arguing that particular *decisions* in particular cases will, or should, be made by the moral philosopher or the lawyer or, as one critic has put it, a 'ghastly on-site Committee'. This would be silly. It is the guidelines for conduct, and the analytical tools, which will be worked out by the non-doctor, along with the doctor. The doctor himself will then have the job of deciding what ought to be done as a matter of good medical ethics in a particular case. He will be left with discretion, which is the right and attraction of all professions. But it is a discretion which is circumscribed, which must be exercised within the limits of generally tolerated conduct. For example, as we have seen, we may never agree on one single proper right course to take in the case of the severely handicapped new-born. But we may decide, for example, that killing by some direct death-dealing action is ethically insupportable and perhaps that slow starvation is equally universally to be avoided. We may establish certain commonly agreed limits within which the doctor must act. The doctor then has the tools with which to decide a particular case. He need no longer substitute his own idiosyncratic sense of right, if by so doing he offends against that which the wider society has indicated is right. So, my message is that those interested in medical ethics come only bearing the offer of help. If doctors were to perceive this, life might be easier and progress made.

In developing good medical ethics, a fundamental rethinking must take place in two particular regards. First, I would put it to you that the Hippocratic tradition is inappropriate now, if it ever were appropriate. I mean by the Hippocratic tradition the notion that the doctor's ethical duty is to the patient before him and to no one else, that the one-to-one relationship marks the boundaries of ethical concern. I suggest that this is inappropriate as a model for a number of reasons. First, it is presented as if it were the only possible ethical way of defining the relationship between doctor and patient, the only possible ethical model. It is not, as I hope to show. By being represented as the only possible ethical model, it is also represented as being the only right one, such that all other models, even if they could be constructed, must by definition be ethically inappropriate. A further objection is that it is a model built on individualism, in which concern for the interests of the group, for the collectivity, if they do not coincide with those of the individual, can properly be ignored. This is expressed in a number of ways. I remind you again of the common claim that the doctor has 'the right to prescribe' to meet the needs of his particular patient, regardless of the implications the exercise of this right may have on the rest. Another objection, which flows from this, is that it allows the doctor to avoid, or shelter from, social responsibility to the collectivity of society, by asserting that *his* responsibility lies only to his patient, an assertion which is self-sustaining and on which the collectivity may not express an opinion since, if you follow the argument, the Hippocratic tradition is, after all, the right, the true model. Then again, it is an inappropriate model in that it is what Robert Veatch, in his paper in the *Hasting Center Report* of June 1972, has called a 'priestly' model, in which the doctor is the benevolent priestly figure, the interpreter of good and bad. This notion is best captured, Veatch suggests, in such expressions as 'speaking as a doctor' when the issue is, for example, the ethics of abortion. A moment's reflection will indicate that being a doctor lends no particular weight to the ethical proposition being advanced.

Good medical ethics, in my view, must provide for a weighing of the interests of the group as well as, and sometimes against, the interests of the individual. There may be some of you to whom talk of regard for collectivism will appear as the rantings of a crypto-Marxist or something rather less polite. Such a reaction would not, I submit, be justified. Indeed, in the everyday practice of medicine, doctors regularly now have to consider the interests of the group, though they may continue to pay lip service to the Hippocratic tradition. Questions concerning the proper allocation of resources among those who could benefit from kidney dialysis is a classic example. *Renal Services*, a report published in July 1982 by two London Regional Health Authorities, shows that, in the United Kingdom, less than half the patients with 'reasonably treatable' kidney failure get treatment. It is particularly patients over 55 years of age who lose out. The consequence is, as Victor Parsons explained in his brilliant short paper in the *Journal of Medical Ethics* of December 1980, that renal units up and down the country have agonizingly to choose which patients will receive dialysis and which will not, and will consequently die. The absence of resources for all means that the patient is seen as a member of a group, each of whom is competing for a scarce resource. And in the competition, as Parsons showed, decisions were made by reference to criteria which may have been expressed and described as medical, but were, in fact, judgements of social merit or worth. Other examples come to mind, such as the ethical decision to inform the parent of the consultation with the 15-year-old girl, or the decision to inform the police of an assault, or to quarantine a patient. And further examples are not hard to find. What I am urging is that good medical ethics will emerge only when this duty to society *as well as* to the particular patient is acknowledged and principles are developed which assist in deciding which duty in the circumstances should prevail.

My final reason for suggesting that the Hippocratic tradition should be abandoned is that as an ethical model it undermines attention to other potentially competing and equally important moral principles. Good medical ethics must embrace these other principles and develop tools for determining which should prevail in given circumstances, if they should conflict. I will make this then my second ground for rethinking medical ethics; the need to incorporate and take account of fundamental moral principles which are largely ignored in the existing approach to medical ethics.

The fundamental principles at present incorporated into traditional medical ethics are those of beneficence and avoiding maleficence, doing good and avoiding harm. Clearly these must continue to be respected but they must not be seen either as the only principles, as is at present the case, or as particularly enlightening as they stand. As regards the latter point, without careful analysis it is not always clear what is good and what is harmful, particularly when the group is considered as against the individual, or when the end in mind is considered rather than the particular present instance. It is not clear, for example, why it is asserted as dogma that it is not for the public good for professionals to criticize a fellow professional. As regards the first point, that they are not the *only* principles, this is what I shall now turn to.

I will offer four basic moral principles which present medical ethics ignores or gives scant attention to, and suggest that good medical ethics must take account of them. In doing so I rely gratefully on the writings of Sisela Bok and Robert Veatch. The first is respect for autonomy. The present 'priestly' model undermines autonomy by suggesting that the doctor is the best and final arbiter of what is good in the practice of medicine. Furthermore, the proposition that the doctor must do good and no harm may conflict with the right to autonomy and may have to give way to it if, for example, the competent patient refuses his consent to further treatment. If, in the exercise of his autonomy, he decides that he does not want good to be done to him, then good medical ethics would suggest that his choice must be respected. At present, with the best will in the world, such a choice is easily undermined, by defining his refusal as evidence of incompetence, so that the doctor or relatives can decide for him, since the doctor views doing good, as defined by the doctor, as the only end to be pursued. The present model of medical ethics allows no proper scope for the exercise of autonomy and the examination of tensions between it and other values.

The second fundamental moral principle is truth-telling and promise-keeping. Here again, the notion of doing good as defined by the professional can work to undermine this moral principle. We have already taken note of the problems associated with informing dying patients of their condition. Now, consider the position of a doctor who works for an industrial company. He may be reluctant to advise a worker who comes to consult him of a symptom which could lead to a slowly debilitating illness. His employers have indicated that if this symptom appears, he should play down its significance. To keep his promise to the company, which is his employer but not his patient, he must conceal the truth from the worker, who is his patient. A solution often suggested is that where a known person's interests are significantly threatened, then this person's interests should prevail. But, of course, this may damage the interests of another known party, the company, and even the rest of the work-force and their dependants, if the company were required to change work practices and could not afford to do so. Perhaps the preferred solution should be that the known physical risk to the employee should outweigh the other speculative, or even real, risks. But once again traditional medical ethics would leave it to the doctor to make this ethical judgement, so that, in truth, the doctor not only claims that trust is at the root of his relationship with his patient, but also claims to be the arbiter of when to observe and when to breach this trust.

The third moral principle which may be ignored in traditional medical ethics is the principle of respect for the dignity of the individual. Once again, a simplistic resort to doing good for the patient may well conflict with respect for his dignity. And a doctor, persuaded that doing good, as defined by him, is the right, indeed the only, principle to follow, will be unable to resolve this conflict except by ignoring the principle of respect for dignity. Thus, for example, we confront the common spectacle of the very old and the very ill languishing in hospital beds, a tribute to the dedication, ingenuity and perseverance of the doctor and his technology, not allowing them to die. Good medical ethics would provide a guide as to when dignity must be respected, even if it means that the doctor must let his patient die. And I interject here that, of course, most doctors are aware of this and do respect this right of the patient to dignity. My point is that it is not formally incorporated into traditional medical ethics.

I have left until last the basic moral principle which I think is the most important and the omission of which from the ambit of current medical ethics I regard as the most serious. This is the principle of seeking to do justice or equity among people. This is the point at which I remind you of my argument that traditional medical ethics is concerned with the individual rather than any regard for the group. Justice or equity may call for consideration of people other than the particular patient; those, for example, who have less access to medical care, or have greater need of it, or those whose health suffers from a misallocation or maldistribution of resources. By claiming that his professional ethic involves concern only for the individual patient, the doctor, like other professionals, can claim to be acting ethically while lamenting the injustices of the system of which he is part. If acting justly, doing justice, were seen to be *the* fundamental moral principle, good medical ethics would clearly mean abandonment of the Hippocratic tradition. Adoption of this principle would, of course, force doctors into taking what may be seen as political stances. They could well be forced to argue that such and such a service − for example, the provision of cardiac care units from which only a few benefit at great cost − cannot and should not be justified, while other services such as the repair of hernias or the provision of sound occupational health measures, which would benefit many at much less cost, were accomplished. And, of course, many doctors may say that such a political stance is not for them; they just want to get on with the job of caring. But this argument cannot be sustained. It ignores the fact that the doctor is *already* taking a political stance by opting for the present state of affairs. It is just as much a political argument to regard doing justice as a problem for others to solve as it is to argue that it is for the profession to become involved in it.

My argument is, therefore, that if the medical profession is to serve, then a new medical ethic, what I have called good medical ethics, must slowly be developed. The principles of autonomy, dignity, justice and partnership must be found a place. The group must be considered as well as the individual. Tools must be developed which give expression to these moral principles and which guide doctors in analysing which principle to respect in an instant case. I believe we have it in our hands to shape a better medical ethic to respond to the dilemmas of modern medicine. There will be some who will react with horror or who will wonder where all this can lead. Will it not destroy the trust at present reposed by the patient in his doctor? I believe it will lead to what we all want: a relationship of *enhanced* trust, a relationship of partners in the enterprise of health in which the moral principles we claim to hold dear enjoy full recognition.

My final question must be, how are we to develop these tools, by which to guide the conduct of doctors. Teaching ethics is not a solution, of course, although it would represent a step forward. We must go further. We are entitled to expect not only some regularity, if not uniformity, in the decisions doctors arrive at, but also some conformity between these decisions and those which the rest of us might make. The principles by reference to which doctors act must be the product of general discussion and debate. They must then be set down in what is thought to be the most appropriate form. There are those who oppose this, or any other form of writing things down. It makes everything appear either to be black and white, they argue, or so grey that you may as well not have bothered. There is some force in this argument, particularly when something as sensitive as caring for someone is involved. But, on balance, it is an argument I reject. The power surrendered to the doctor, the freedom and responsibility abandoned by the individual, if the appropriate principles are not laid down, are too great. They outweigh any anxieties over the problems drawing up a set of rules or guidelines may pose. There must be a framework of rules. Indeed, they exist already as regards many areas of practice. But in some cases they are not clear and in others developments have proceeded at such a pace that we have not really had time adequately to take them in and suggest how they be resolved. The question becomes, then, what form this framework of rules of conduct should take. This is the practical issue.

What options are available? We can discount leaving it to the individual doctor to draw up his own rules or to the medical profession as a group. These matters are for all of us, though, of course, the doctor has an important role to play, not only in educating us as to the facts involved, but also the consequences and practicality of particular proposals. One framework of rules is already with us. In many situations, we must refer to the law. It already stipulates how the doctor is to act. You may ask, what has law to do with medical ethics? Well, if ethics concerns what ought or ought not to be done in given circumstances, given the goals to be achieved, obviously ethics is going to overlap the law. Law has the same concern, that of regulating human conduct and affairs according to agreed principles and rules. Many ethical problems also have legal implications. This is because we, as a society, take certain conduct sufficiently seriously that we choose to regulate it by the use of law, backed ultimately by the threat of force to be used against those who disobey. Other conduct may not be regarded as warranting recourse to the heavy armoury, the siege-gun, of the law. We may, instead, be content to rely on sanctions other than force, such as social pressure, disapproval, censure or ostracism, or on an individual's conscience. For example, whether you ought to cheat when playing cards with your neighbours or when filling in your tax return involves a consideration of ethics. Specifically, it involves the ethical principle that you ought ordinarily to tell the truth. But one of the two questions also involves the law, since, while society can leave cheating at cards to other sanctions, it takes cheating the Revenue seriously enough to have laws against it.

This overlap between ethics and law exists in the field of medical practice just as elsewhere. Questions such as whether a doctor ought to expose an elderly female patient to the gaze of all, while examining her in a hospital ward, or whether he ought to treat her with drugs despite her refusal, are both to be answered by reference to ethical principles. In particular, they invoke consideration of the ethical principle of respect for the dignity of another. The answer to the second question also calls for consideration of the law. There is a point in the behaviour of one person to another beyond which it is not thought sufficient to leave the matter to conscience or some disorganized informal sanctions.

When both ethics and law are involved in regulating medical practice, it is essential that they agree. Good law should reflect and promote good medical ethics. Law which is ethically unsound will soon lose respect and deservedly so. We all know, of course, the disadvantages of having law involved, whether it be the product of Parliament or the courts. It is often a heavy-handed way of dealing with a problem and this is as true of medical practice as it is of, for example, labour relations or race relations. The feeling is that without hard and fast rules and the threat of formal sanctions, without the heat of adversarial argument, sensitive and delicate matters could be managed in an appropriately sensitive, humane and flexible way.

That said, the plain fact of the matter is that the law, as we have seen, is involved. Indeed, there are few areas of medical practice not regulated by law as well as ethics. Thus, it is no good arguing, as do some, that the law has no place in the operating or consulting room, that medical practice is too complex or too private an area for law. The law is already there, like it or not. Think back, if you will, to the problems associated with the treatment of the severely handicapped new-born baby. The fact is that we are talking about whether a child lives or dies, how a doctor ought to behave, what his duty is. This inevitably means that the law is involved. The State takes very seriously conduct which is life-threatening; sufficiently seriously to outlaw it, to make it a crime in most cases. Quite properly it demands that when a doctor has a child in his care and allows it to die, he provide some good justification. Quite properly, it puts him to proof that his conduct meets the standards of behaviour which we as a society, through our law, judge to be appropriate. Quite properly, such a question is not left to individual conscience or social disapproval, since the life of another, the child, is involved. As *The Times* pointed out, in its editorial of 6 November 1981, 'It is, of course, parents and doctors on whom it falls to take these agonizing decisions in the first place, and they deserve the understanding and support of society. But they are decisions of a kind that are required to be taken inside a framework of public morality which finds its expression and sanction in the law.'

Of course, if the law is involved, we are entitled to hope that it will be good law, that it will reflect good medical ethics. Doctors too are equally entitled to law which will guide them, but not require them to do that which makes no sense in terms of good medical practice and care. Law which results from criminal prosecutions, as in the case of Dr Arthur, or hastily convened hearings, as in the case of *Re B*, may not always meet these standards. Granted the law must speak, or be made to speak, on questions such as the proper treatment of the new-born. But, you may ask, are there not better ways of getting legal guidance? To the extent that we think that the law is poor or unclear, one response could be to seek to change or clarify the law through taking a case to court or pressing for legislation. Given the pressure of time on Parliament, legislation ought, perhaps, to be reserved for major issues of social policy on which there may be a strong division of view, and what is needed is a general framework for the future. The Abortion Act or the Mental Health Act are examples. Legislation is not for piecemeal solution of specific issues. But what of litigation? I am not persuaded that this is a particularly fruitful exercise. One of the rare circumstances in which it might be called for is where the law is unclear and this lack of clarity may serve as a deterrent, preventing those who wish to act in what is generally regarded as a proper way from doing so. But, in such circumstances, it is quite wrong that the law should have to be tested or developed by bringing a civil claim, or, worse, a prosecution. Civil suits depend on the coming together of a person with time, money, energy and perseverance, and a claim which can stand up on its facts and in terms of its merit. To leave the development of the law to such a happy coincidence of factors is to guarantee it goes undeveloped. To pillory in the dock, in a criminal prosecution, someone who may well have thought that his conduct was entirely justifiable, is even less satisfactory, particularly since it is often difficult in the extreme in a jury trial to dig out what law has emerged as distinct from what the verdict was.

Unfortunately, these are the only ways we have, effectively, of changing our law. It must be a task for the future to persuade Parliament or the courts to come up with more suitable ways of testing or finding out the law. It has to be said that we, in England, have been less than imaginative in our ways of shaping the law. This is particularly so as regards medical law, where guidance is sorely needed and, as long as the law is not clear, it is always open to some individual or group to appear from the woodwork and press some prosecution or law suit. One method, largely unused and worthy of much greater expansion, is the petition for a declaratory judgment. The court is asked to declare what the law is on given facts. This is a device much used, and with great success, in the United States. It avoids the situation which prevails at present in England, in which the only way to discover whether what you intend is lawful is to do it and then wait to see whether anyone sues or prosecutes and if so, whether the court decides in your favour. This is the kind of muddling approach which Jeremy Bentham once castigated as waiting until the dog bites and then kicking it. Clearly, when modern medical practice is throwing up hosts of deeply troubling problems, this is a less than satisfactory way to proceed.

Ironically, on the question of the treatment of the severely handicapped new-born, developments in the United States have not taken their usual course. Certainly cases have been taken to court, hospital ethics committees have deliberated, State legislatures have debated and the President's Commission for the Study of Ethical Problems in Medicine held meetings in June 1982 with a view to drafting an appropriate set of guidelines. This is the response which can be expected where the issue is one which divides communities and has to be seen against the backdrop of the Constitutional protection of life and the political values of the New Right. What was unexpected and perhaps a response to this political constituency was the decision of the Secretary at the Department of Health and Human Resources, Richard Schweiker. In early 1982 he sent a letter to some 6,000 hospitals advising the administrators that to withhold treatment from handicapped new-borns was against Federal law. There is no Federal law of murder or manslaughter, apart from circumstances such as hijacking aeroplanes. The law he referred to was the 1973 Rehabilitation Act, which had not previously been regarded as crucial in this area. It is unlikely that this rather heavy-handed approach has aided deliberation or made a sensitive answer more readily attainable.

The way to avoid legislation or litigation is to draw up rules or guidelines in the form of a Code of Practice. I do not see such a Code (or Codes) as needing to be passed into law. It would be in such a form as to indicate that if a doctor complied with it then his conduct could properly be regarded as ethical and lawful. If he deviated from it, this would be good evidence of unethical and unlawful conduct unless a sufficiently good reason could be given. Codes of Practice are not novelties. We already make considerable use of them in labour relations and in commercial affairs. There are already a number of Codes of Practice in medicine also. We have Codes regulating such matters as transplantation surgery, the determination of death, and experimentation and medical research. And their value is not limited to ethical problems in which the law is involved. They would be of equal, if not more, value in areas in which the law is not involved (and in which, as a consequence, there may be even less clear a guide at present), expressing the view of the community as to the appropriate conduct to be followed, and serving as a guide for the doctor.

Against the background of all this talk of regulation, the doctor may well ask what benefit, if any, would flow to him from the drawing up of a Code of Practice. My answer, put shortly, is that it would provide the basis for a relationship of partners in which trust can exist. The Code would only help the doctor, though, tragically, there are many doctors who fail, or refuse, to perceive this. It would help in that the doctor would be able to look to the Code for guidance and analysis. It would help in that the doctor could point to it by way of explaining his actions to his patient. Taking this time and effort to communicate, and having some authoritative guide to point to, would be of incalculable benefit in fostering good doctor–patient relations. It would help the doctor to be a good doctor. He is a moral agent. No longer would he have to mask the real nature of his decisions or rely on some visceral sense of what is right, only to be criticized whatever he does. Finally, it would help the patient and the community, not only by creating the basis for trust, but also by serving as the basis on which to judge and, if appropriate, criticize the doctor's actions.

It only remains to ask, who would draw up such a Code of Practice? Experience in the United Kingdom demonstrates that, in the odd cases in which Codes exist, the British Medical Association has taken it as its prerogative, or specialist groups, consisting in the past largely of doctors, have been convened to respond to a particular problem, only to be disbanded once their report is presented or the Code is drafted. There are, for example, three groups, from the British Medical Association, the Royal College of Obstetricians and Gynaecologists and the Council on Science and Society, all now considering separately the ethical implications arising from research into and the practice of *in vitro* fertilization. 'Inquiries into the issues raised by new medical techniques of human reproduction are proliferating', said *The Times* editorial of 19 April 1982. 'It is no disparagement to the organizations setting out to make their own contributions to the debate', it went on, 'to say that they cannot be an adequate substitute for an authoritative and wide-ranging public inquiry.' As if in response to this and other such expressions of opinion, the DHSS announced in July 1982 the establishment of a fourth working party.

This *ad hoc* response, knocking off problems when the public pressure for action makes it politic to do so, is less than satisfactory, though better than no response at all. It tends to dissipate the energies, expertise and experience of those involved. It allows for no continuity or coherence of analysis or experience. It atomizes medical ethics into discrete problems and thereby creates the danger that the interaction of issues and values across the broad spectrum of medical practice will be overlooked or given less than appropriate consideration.

The most appropriate course lies in the creation by Parliament or the DHSS of a Permanent Standing Advisory Committee charged with the task of drawing up Codes of Practice and of keeping developments in medicine under constant review, with a view to identifying and responding to ethical issues. It would have a permanent secretariat. It would hear evidence, issue working papers, invite comments and, then, draft Codes. A similar institution already exists in the form of the Law Commission, which is charged with keeping the state of the law under review and proposing draft legislation where appropriate, after proper consultation. The aim of the Advisory Committee should be slowly to produce a comprehensive Code of Practice governing the ethics of medical practice. The secretariat would consist of specialists in such disciplines as medicine, ethics, law and economics. The members of the Committee would be drawn from representatives of appropriate constituencies, and be responsible to Parliament or the appropriate Minister. Doctors, medical scientists, other health professionals, priests and theologians, and representatives of industry and labour would all be likely members. A precedent for such a body already exists in the President's Commission for the Study of Ethical Problems in Medicine and Biomedical and Behavioral Research, which has functioned successfully in the United States since 1976. We could well follow the example, though not perhaps the title! The activities of the Australian Law Reform Commission in the field of medical law and ethics under its distinguished Chairman, Mr Justice Kirby, also serve as an example for us of energy, sensitive analysis and practical solutions.

I have reviewed decision-making in medicine, choosing some specific examples to make my points. I have examined what medical ethics is about. I have suggested ways we can inch our way towards solving what are extremely difficult problems. We must find a way for the future. We must face up to and resolve these hard moral problems of modern medicine. We must ignore the overweening hubris of those members of the medical profession who would deny us the opportunity to do so. We owe it to our doctors and to ourselves.

5 The doors of mental illness

George says he is going to kill himself. What should we do? Should we express concern? Should we do more and, if so, what more? Is George ill? Is George mentally ill? Bill believes, quite wrongly, that the Inland Revenue is pursuing a vendetta against him. He leaves home and family and begins to wander around, living rough. What should we do? Should we try to persuade him to see someone and, if so, whom should he see? And if he says no, what then? Is Bill ill? Is Bill mentally ill? Tom believes that this country's problems will be solved only if immigrants from the new Commonwealth countries are caused to leave. He makes speeches regularly and publishes a monthly newsletter which pursues this theme. What should we do about Tom? Is he ill? Is Tom mentally ill?

These questions are among the more taxing we face in our modern society. Any answers must draw on our sense of right and wrong, of propriety, of normality, of order, of law and authority, and perhaps, most significant, our sense of freedom and responsibility. At what point does caring become controlling? At what point does freedom become dangerous? This, to me, is what is involved in any examination of mental illness. As I search for an answer, keep in mind that these are practical problems. Keep in mind that the easiest solution, at least superficially, is to 'put people away', as the expression goes. This has a fine historical precedent. To what extent we can, or should, continue to do it is a question which will dog us throughout. Keep in mind that my concern from the outset has been with the twin notions of responsibility and power, in the context of the practice of medicine. Nowhere are these notions more clearly involved than in the context of mental illness. To be judged mentally ill is to be judged, to a greater or lesser extent, not responsible. The implications for freedom and its denial are profound. You only get your life back when others judge you responsible again.

Any consideration of mental illness must take as its starting-point the question 'What is mental illness?' It is common knowledge that there are some who argue vehemently that mental illness is, in the words of the most famous polemicist, Thomas Szasz, a myth. He has it that the notion of mental illness exists as a mechanism for social control, for medicalizing, medicating, even incarcerating those regarded as social misfits. It represents a conspiracy between us and the specialist, the expert. It looks respectable if the expert does it, whereas we would feel uncomfortable, or even guilty, if we used other social means to achieve the object desired. And, Szasz seems to argue, we have created a monster. The power, once granted to experts, cannot be taken away. So we stumble along and hope not too much harm is done.

Of course, Szasz does not go unanswered. Psychiatrists, psychologists, analysts and laymen line up regularly to shoot at him, each one delivering what he sees as the *coup de grâce*. They dispute the very basis of his objection to mental illness, so it is as well to recall what this is. The principal point made by Szasz is that the word 'illness' is properly applied to physical illness, where a disease entity exists. No such physical disease entity exists in the case of mental illness, therefore it cannot be called illness. It is, instead, a moral or political judgement. But this argument is fundamentally flawed. The flaw does not lie in the point that there are, in fact, disease entities in the case of mental illness. Rather, the flaw lies in the failure to understand that illness, in the form of alleged physical illness, is equally a normative or judgemental term. Illness is more than the existence of a set of objective conditions. It is a judgement that a particular status, that of being ill, ought to be ascribed to someone in whom those conditions are present. Depending on the judgement made, the doctor grants or withholds the status. So there is no reason in principle why the notion of illness should be restricted to physical states. It can just as well be extended to thoughts, mood or behaviour. If it is decided that these warrant the evaluative judgement that they should be regarded as illness, then illness they can be. Equally, in principle, for want of a better term, they can be called mental illness. Thus, in short, the intellectual basis for Szasz's argument is misconceived. It is not a telling argument to say, as does Szasz, that there is no such thing as mental illness, since illness is not a thing. Despite this flaw, however, the insight and observations of Szasz remain valuable. He asks the right questions even if for the wrong reason. For what has to be considered is whether the judgemental term 'illness' should be used in the way it is.

Before going on, perhaps I ought to respond to the arguments of those who say that there are specific disease entities and conditions, which amount to mental illness. Certainly, having accepted the notion of mental illness into our culture, you can see how our language reflects the imagery of disease. We speak of someone as 'having a screw loose', of being 'not quite all there', or, in American argot, of 'losing his marbles'. All of these are obviously mechanistic explanations. We resort to them because we do not have any persuasive non-materialist analogy to capture what we want to convey. We are after all trying to describe something which, in our hearts, we suspect is a judgement on someone, that he is odd, or different, or should be treated differently, or cared for, or should be avoided. There are, for example, those who regard the mind as being the product of the complex biochemistry of the brain. At least for them, the day may soon dawn when we can relate mental qualities and attributes to the brain's biochemistry. They would deduce from this the dramatic assertion that mental illness will then be shown, in fact, to be mere biochemical malfunctioning. Mental illness will then be just another form of physical illness.

Things are not so easy. This materialist way out is hopelessly flawed. Notice the circularity in the argument that mental illness is biochemical malfunctioning. It begs the question. It assumes what has to be proved: that certain particular mental states, ways of thinking, moods, behaviour, temperament, ought to be regarded as illnesses. Only when we agree that they ought to be so regarded will any biochemical abnormality be relevant. Equally, until we do agree which mental states should be regarded as illnesses, biochemistry is unimportant. For there are, of course, numerous biochemical deviations from a notional norm in all of us. Most will not be regarded as indicative of illness. Only those correlating most closely with behaviour we have already decided to categorize as mentally ill will be selected. Those who look to biochemistry, therefore, have the cart very firmly before the horse.

To those who do not sail under this flag, the mind is more than its biochemistry, though what more, and how so, is not readily clear. Denying that the mind is completely to be understood in terms of material substance, it is not readily open to them to describe mental illness in terms of diseased parts. Ultimately, they are forced to fall back on the notion of disease by analogy, as indicating a deviation from the norm which, if it were in the context of the physical body, would be called a disease. When even the notion of disease by analogy seems too strong, or causes momentary intellectual misgivings, you see the term 'mental disorder' being used, conveying the notion that whatever the proper order is, or ought to be, this person's mental order is not.

So I regard the disease approach to mental illness as untenable. This is not to say that mental illness is a myth, merely that the efforts of those engaged in practising the arcane skills of mental health care to defend it on materialist grounds seem insupportable. Of course, we should note in passing that this does not seem to have threatened in any way the continued claim to recognition of mental illness. Whatever the route taken, the architects of mental illness have created an edifice, similar in size and structure to that of their colleagues in the field of physical illness. Diseases have been noted. Taxonomical skills have broken them down by genus, species, and sub-species. Specialists and sub-specialists have arisen to meet the need created by a new species or sub-species, and then, most important, people have been found who are suffering from a particular illness or disease. I have not inverted the natural course of events. I think it eminently arguable that, in the case of mental illness, the experts and categorizers came first, the people to fill the categories later, just as the buildings to house them came first. As Michel Foucault argues in his book *Madness and Civilisation*, the emptying of the lazar houses of lepers was followed by the filling of them with those who would now be called the mentally ill.

So is there a better way of understanding mental illness? The key, of course, lies in its counterpart, mental health. Just as with other notions of health, a norm is involved. In this case, it is the norm of thinking, of behaviour, mood or feeling. To describe someone as mentally ill represents a judgement that his thinking, or mentation, mood, behaviour or feeling, deviates sufficiently from the norm to warrant ascribing the status 'ill' to him. And there you have the dilemma of mental illness. As a notion, it is unmanageable. If, in the case of purported physical illness, it was difficult to map out the limits and bounds of the appropriate use of the concept of illness, it is that much more difficult in the case of mental illness. Yet map them out we must. For what is at stake is a concern for each person's liberty and self-determination.

It is imperative that the power of the expert to use the label 'mentally ill' not go unsupervised. But there seems no ready limit to its use, it is such a will-o'-the-wisp. At least in the case of physical illness, though it is a judgemental term, it is a judgement made in the light of the presence of some physical condition. This gives some guide, albeit very rudimentary, to the proper use and meaning of the term. But the very immateriality of mental illness, its other-worldliness, its association with the subjective world of the mind, rather than any physical state, deprives us of even this guide to the limit of its proper use.

So each time we challenge the use of the term 'mental illness' in a particular case there is no ready guide or boundary to point to, so as to show that the particular application of the term is inappropriate or unjustified. We are forced to challenge the very basis of the concept, to deny its validity, or to say that even if it is valid as a notion we do not think it should be applied to the particular case before us. But the entrenched power of those who manipulate the concept of mental illness and the fact that they have boot-strapped themselves into intellectual respectability serve to defeat such challenges. 'If you do not believe in mental illness, what more can we say?' It may appear a weak argument, but our ready acceptance of the authority of the community of experts and their willingness, indeed desire, to use their power for their own continued existence allow it to carry the day. Equally, to say that George or Bill or Tom is not, in your opinion, mentally ill is to be met by such ready responses as 'What do you know about it?' or 'As experts, we think otherwise.' Again the power of the expert, rather than the power of the argument, defeats the challenge. Thus, intellectually and conceptually, there are no ready limits, no rationally defensible borders, to the notion of mental illness. It is a question of accepting the whole package or being thought a fool or a rabble-rouser. The implication, of course, is that we forfeit the right and ability to question the manipulation of the notion, the propriety of its attribution to George, or Bill or Tom. All the power lies with the expert, and we must just hope and trust.

As I have said, someone is deemed mentally ill when he deviates from the appropriate norm of mental health. Let us now concentrate on this norm for a while. By so doing, I shall attempt to explain how someone comes to be categorized as mentally ill. There are, in fact, two steps. The first involves a determination that George's thoughts, or moods, are abnormal. The second entails a further judgement, the nature of which is most elusive. It has something to do with how important, and I choose a vague term at this stage, how important the abnormality is.

Consider the first step. To ask the question 'What are normal thoughts?' is to expose the nature of the enterprise. Heaven alone knows what thoughts all of us harbour, or have harboured, in our time. If the norm were a composite of the thoughts and moods of all of us who confidently assert we are not mentally ill, then the norm would have no meaning, because it would embrace just about everything susceptible to being thought. So it has to be something different. It has to be a norm based on what we think people should think or feel, a standard we set for ourselves, though we may not keep it. Stated in this fashion, it can be seen that the norm involved is a moral or social or political one. It is a composite of the right moral, social and political thoughts. So as not to throw the baby out with the bath-water, I will concede that there may be near-universal agreement that certain thoughts are wrong. For example, for me to think that walking naked through the streets of London is socially appropriate would be wrong. But, even if we accept that this is wrong, there is other conduct about which there would not be near-universal agreement as to its rightness or wrongness, and, of course, near-universal agreement is only a satisfactory criterion of what is right provided you accept the principle of right by numbers. So, even at this first stage, we grant power to those claiming expertise to make moral, social or political judgements about the rightness of someone's thoughts, or mood, or feeling, or behaviour. Of course, to say that one must think right thoughts or run the risk of being labelled mentally ill is to conjure up the image of *Nineteen Eighty-Four*, or of the Soviet Union, or some other nasty place. But, unwrapped from its package of expertise, and what some have mischievously christened psychobabble, this is what you have here in your midst — more subtle, yes, and less oppressive in the fact, perhaps, but still the same.

The second step is then involved. Your thoughts are abnormal, wrong. But is the abnormality important enough to warrant invoking the judgement 'mental illness'? What does 'important' mean here? This is, of course, at the heart of any discussion of mental health. There are two elements in my notion of importance: that which is so threatening that it goes beyond what we are prepared to tolerate, and that which evokes a particular kind of sympathy, in that the expert involved would wish paternalistically and, perhaps, patronizingly to do something. These two elements are eminently flexible and vague, even though they are so significant. Different things threaten different people. Equally, our view of those who need and deserve help may vary with the fashions of the day. As David Ingleby argues, in his paper *The Social Construction of Mental Illness*, 'seeing someone's point of view involves a minimal degree of willingness to share that point of view . . . understanding someone is simply not possible without crediting them with a basic degree of plausibility'. If the thoughts or mood or behaviour already judged to be abnormal and therefore wrong are, on these tests, also judged to be importantly wrong, then the process of segregating someone as mentally ill is set in motion. The first step is to take control over the person, because to be mentally ill is to be out of control. Usually, the very act of diagnosing him as mentally ill is sufficient to allow the expert to gain control. If any doubt arises, we are, of course, always ready to support the expert in his view. Once he is controlled, by being labelled, and thereby under the power of the expert, the question of what response should be made − what should be done with, or to, the person − can be duly considered.

The implications of this process are clear. We have chosen to allow the coming into being of a group of people who claim an expertise in mental health, or right thinking. We have chosen to allow them to apply the status 'ill' to those of our fellow men whose thoughts, or words, or behaviour, do not pass muster. We have done this knowing that the nature of the expertise is in reality the exercise of moral, social and political judgement concerning the worth of someone's thinking. We must realize that this power, once granted, is not easily taken away. But we have slept easily in our beds, secure in the knowledge that, here at least, the power is not abused. Only those whom we would all regard as having really abnormal thoughts and posing a real threat, or being really in need of care, have attracted the status 'mentally ill'.

The reality may not conform to this cosy image. One-third of hospital beds are occupied by those categorized as mentally ill. One in eight or nine of us will, at some time in his life, be diagnosed as suffering from mental illness. Five million people in England consult their family doctors each year about their mental health. Six hundred thousand are referred to specialist psychiatric services. There are 21,000 cases each year of compulsory detention in mental hospitals. Some have spoken of an epidemic of mental illness. Is it that the experts are being a little too zealous, seeing mental illness around every corner, spotting threatening thoughts, and people needing help with their thoughts, at every turn, or are there other explanations?

The explanation I offer is that two contradictory patterns of behaviour can be seen. On the one hand, large numbers of people seek the refuge of the status 'ill'. To be classified as ill is to be excused of everyday responsibility, to be treated like a child. Lacking the faith that fortified their predecessors, they turn to the new religion of mental illness, in which they may confess and hope to be absolved, as painlessly as possible, by the expert. The stigma of being categorized as mentally ill is, of course, still with us, though less pronounced. But to some it may be a price worth paying for the refuge they seek.

On the other hand, while some may choose it, others may have the status forced upon them. They, too, find the pressures of our harsh world insupportable. They are not limited to those who meta-phorically crack from these pressures. They may well include, depending on the nature of the society at the time, those who do not, or will not, fit. A successful, open and confident society tolerates wide variations in thought and behaviour. A society under stress becomes less tolerant. The forces of law become more vigilant or oppressive, depending on the view taken. But the process is not limited to the forces of law. Others involved in the maintenance of the prevailing social values are pressed into aid. Mental illness experts are among them. Political differences can become deviance, a code word on occasions for illness. Social protest can become irrational and dangerous behaviour. The black man who makes a speech calling for the destruction of the 'white devils' will be 'remanded for a psychiatric report'. Sexual predilections can become sick depravities. We begin to use madness as a metaphor for those things we disapprove of in our society. Suddenly, the metaphor takes on a life of its own. That which was metaphor now becomes illness. The doors of mental illness are cranked open to receive new classes of wrong thinkers. The expert becomes society's agent, the socializer, even, on occasions, the thought policeman.

The similarity between the processes of criminal law and the resort to the notion of mental illness are clear, but the crucial distinction is that the criminal law does not prohibit mere thoughts, nor does it reach a verdict without trial and the right to appeal. Indeed, it is salutary to notice the inter-relationship between the criminal law and mental illness. Much that is deemed immoral in our society is punished by the criminal law, but some immoral conduct is not prohibited, even though it is not necessarily approved of. The reason may be that there is sufficient disagreement about its immorality or otherwise to make the passing of legislation difficult or counter-productive.

But this is not the end of the story. There is still the possibility that anyone engaged in, or even contemplating, this immoral conduct may be judged both wrong-thinking and a threat. If this be the case, he can always be categorized as mentally ill, and thereby dealt with just as effectively. Let me offer just one example. Consider the man who thinks about — indeed, let us go further, plans on his own — the killing of an enemy. He is guilty of no crime, even if his intentions or plans become known. Nor would he ordinarily be judged, in our society, to be mentally ill. Only if he were to carry out his plan would he be at risk, and then it would be before the criminal courts, where he could speak for himself and offer what defence he thought fitting. By contrast, consider the man who thinks of having some sort of sexual contact with a young girl, let us say aged ten, or with a young boy of the same age, and makes plans to carry this out. Should these plans or thoughts become known, he is greatly at risk of being caught in the web of mental illness. He does not have to carry out his plan, the thoughts are enough. They may not be thought to be more threaten-ing or dangerous than those of the man with homicide on his mind. Yet one may acquire the status 'mentally ill', the other not. And more, once he is diagnosed, or fixed with the label 'mentally ill', his liberty and future life become something for others to dispose of, while our homicidal friend walks free.

In between these two groups are the mass of mentally ill — un-happy, awkward, social misfits, who neither volunteer themselves for mental illness nor attract the status of mentally ill because of their threatening ways. By their conduct, by their inability to cope, by their position on the outskirts of our reality, they are noticed, and it is decided that something ought to be done.

What I have sought to do so far is to demonstrate the shaky intellectual basis on which the concept of mental illness rests. It follows that very great caution must be exercised in visiting the status of mentally ill upon someone. I am aware that the reply could come back that the precise borders between mental illness and mental health may be hard to draw, but, in a particular case, it is usually not hard to see on which side of the line they are. To use an analogy, red and purple shade together, but we still have no difficulty, the argument goes, in differentiating crimson from royal purple. The medievalists encapsulated this idea by stating that there was no difficulty in identifying what was horse and what was tail, though it may not be clear when the horse begins and the tail ends. Thus, is it not open to those involved with mental illness to concede some of the definitional difficulties I have alluded to, yet still insist on the validity of their notion of mental illness? Mr Smith's habit, for example, of washing his hands repeatedly, so causing him anguish and virtually paralysing his existence, would, they may argue, fall clearly into the category of mentally ill, as it would if he thought himself to be a messenger from heaven with a divine mission to kill prostitutes and was intent on beginning the job.

There are at least two responses to this argument. One, the more radical, is not one I favour, though it is respectable as a thesis. According to it, we can admit that Mr Smith is behaving or thinking in an abnormal way. We can admit that he should attract concern and care. But, thereafter, we can say that the argument we have heard has a quality of self-validation about it. For it does not follow that Mr Smith should be regarded as ill. He is different. His difference causes him anguish. But to call him ill is to cause certain consequences to flow which are not necessarily entailed by his condition. This is because illness is not a descriptive term, but one which only has meaning within a larger system of ideas, language and values. Illness is an abstraction. To call Mr Smith mentally ill only carries the necessary significance or meaning if it is understood within a system of ideas and assumptions about the mind, behaviour, normality and illness. And, of course, it is these assumptions and ideas, this system of reasoning, of which we are not convinced.

So, this more radical response goes on, it is not as simple to say Mr Smith is clearly mentally ill as it is to say this colour is clearly crimson. We all agree as a matter of convention that crimson shall be used to describe a particular shade of red. We all agree that Mr Smith is clearly in a separate category, in terms of his behaviour or thinking, from, say, Mr Jones, whose thinking and behaviour are normal. But we do not necessarily agree that Mr Smith's category should be called mental illness. All we have agreed is that it is different. But difference does not connote illness. We want to know what else there is that makes him mentally ill. To describe him as mentally ill channels Mr

Smith down a certain path. It tends to foreclose other ways of regarding him. It causes caring to be translated into treating. It means that caring becomes a specialist matter to be placed in the hands of experts. That is what the word treatment implies. This is what calling him mentally ill implies.

An alternative response to the crimson–purple, horse–tail argument, which is less radical and the one I endorse, is as follows. Let us accept that Mr Smith falls clearly into an identifiably different category. Let us even call this mental illness. My only aim has been to point to the difficulties inherent in drawing the necessary boundaries between mental illness and mental health. Too much seems to me to be neither crimson nor purple. Furthermore, what was purple, in the realm of mental illness, has a habit of becoming crimson with disconcerting ease. This is because, as I have said, illness is not a descriptive term, applied, as is crimson, to some objective reality. We cannot properly differ as to whether something is crimson in the realm of colours. We can as to whether someone is mentally ill. Specialists do so all the time! This vagueness, and the implicit values and assumptions which underlie it, have to be considered in the context of the consequences of describing Mr Smith as mentally ill. Not the least of these is the undermining of his power over, and responsibility for, his own destiny.

Thus, my argument becomes, as I have said already, that we must use the greatest care in describing someone as mentally ill. We must be aware of the intellectual baggage such a description brings with it. We must exercise appropriate control over its use. We are entitled to expect a clearer spectrum which allows us to identify something we would all be prepared to call crimson. We are entitled to an analysis of mental illness which addresses itself more carefully to why we use the term, what function we seek to make it serve. Perhaps, by using the analogy of a legal contract, I can make this last and most important point in the clearest way. No analysis of the word contract is of any real value unless it takes account of the function the notion of contract is supposed to serve. Fundamentally, it is used to identify bargains or agreements which parties ought to be held to, on threat of some sanction, such that if one renegues on his part of the bargain he can be made to compensate the other. With this insight, the law of contract can be properly understood, and the particular rules shaped so as to serve this primary function through changing times. When two parties fall out over a bargain, the fruitful question is not, is their bargain a contract, but rather, is their bargain one to which the word contract ought to apply, with all the consequences which flow from this?

This is the analysis which should attend consideration of mental illness. We should ask what purpose we seek to achieve by using the term. We should then ask whether that purpose is served by describing Mr Smith as mentally ill. And the only purpose it may properly have is to serve as a means of caring and helping in ways which cannot otherwise be achieved, and by people who are uniquely equipped to do so.

The implications of being categorized as mentally ill, both in terms of the freedom and responsibility of the individual and in terms of the power of the professional, cannot be overstated. This is particularly true in those circumstances in which we go so far as to sanction the compulsory detention in hospitals of certain groups of those classified as mentally ill. You will recall that there are 21,000 cases of compulsory admission to hospital in England every year. And, of course, there are many more who are voluntarily in hospital, but who, doubtless, would be detained under the law if they tried to leave. They may then be subjected to treatment without their consent, and lose most of the freedoms and rights associated with citizenship, for example voting (subject to recent decisions of the English and Scottish courts), taking a matter to court, spending money or making a will. It is hardly surprising that the idea of compulsory detention of the mentally ill attracts the greatest concern. The grounds on which a person may be detained are still, at the present moment, set out in the 1959 Mental Health Act. They are ill defined, as befits anything concerned with mental illness. Someone may be compulsorily admitted if two medical practitioners are prepared to recommend it. In cases deemed emergencies, only one medical recommendation is needed. The person has to be suffering from a 'mental disorder', which is defined, if that be the correct word, to include 'mental illness', 'severe subnormality', or 'psychopathic disorder'. Then the disorder has to be 'of a nature and degree which justifies detention', and it must be 'in the interest of his health or safety or for the protection of others' that he should be detained. That someone's liberty should rest on such flimsy criteria, and the say-so of someone claiming expertise, is startling.

I referred, just now, to the grounds for detention *at the present moment.* This is because, after numerous efforts and recommendations for change, new law will appear on the statute book in the autumn of 1982, in the form of the Mental Health (Amendment) Act. This is the first Parliamentary review of the law for twenty-three years and its drafting and passage through Parliament have seen some spirited debate and no little disagreement. Here is not the place to attempt any exegesis of the proposed law, particularly as it is still in the process of being written as it rumbles between Lords and Commons. But I can offer some general comments.

My principal concern with the proposed new law is as someone concerned about the civil liberties and freedoms of individuals categorized as mentally ill. The question, then, for me, is the extent to which this law meets objections which have previously been made. The answer is that there are some considerable improvements and some disappointments. This is, of course, the nature of law-making. It is inevitable. What improvements there are arise in no small part from the efforts of Mind, the National Association for Mental Health, and, in particular, its indefatigable and immensely able legal director, Larry Gostin. No other person has done more, or as much, to keep the civil libertarian's concerns and arguments before the legislators' minds. The disappointments are discouraging, and because, as I shall suggest, they relate to such crucial areas, they are much to be regretted.

One of the most important changes, in the context of compulsory detention, is the acceptance of the notion of treatability; that, in essence, someone may not be detained unless his condition is one which is amenable to treatment. This means that the mental hospital will not be as readily available in the future as a dumping ground for the awkward and unwanted. Indeed, those already confined as long-stay patients will also benefit, since there will now be an automatic right to review for anyone detained for more than three years. It also means that ways will have to be found of adequately caring for, and about, such people as they live among us in the community. Equally important are the improvements in the machinery for reviewing detention, for dealing with complaints and conditions, in the shortening of the periods of time during which a person may be detained before review, and in the development of special rules as regards certain types of controversial treatment, such as electro-convulsive therapy, long-term drug use and psychosurgery.

There are two principal areas of disappointment. They are in the consideration of the definition of mental illness, and the proposals concerned with consent to treatment. With the concept of treatability, these are at the root of any concern for the liberty and dignity of the individual. All other changes are contingent upon this fundamental structure, so that if it is not sound, they lose much of their force and significance. The improvement reflected in the adoption of treatability is greatly diminished by the decisions taken in the other two areas. The provisions defining mental illness remain quite unjustifiably vague. The language remains the same, except that the notion of 'subnormality' has been replaced by 'mental impairment'. The grounds for detention also remain the same. As regards consent to treatment, it should be noted that the 1959 Act is completely silent on this matter. So it was no small improvement to have the legal position spelled out in particular provisions. But, on the whole, the result is less than satisfactory, save for the provision which states that certain kinds of treatment, which are the subject of controversy, may not under any circumstances be performed without a patient's consent. This is a most important step.

Otherwise, the question is, under what circumstances may a mentally ill person be treated without his consent. It was conceded by all that treatment without consent was justified in certain circumstances. Issue was joined, however, over whether there should be review of any decision to treat without consent, to ensure that in the particular circumstances it was, in fact, appropriate. The issue was, in other words, whether any second opinion should be sought. And, even if the notion of review were to be accepted in principle, the question remained, who should do the reviewing? The position of Mind, and others, was that review was called for in all cases of treatment without consent, and that the review should be by persons other than doctors. The Royal College of Psychiatrists was not persuaded. The need for consent, and a review of this consent to ensure that it was freely given, were grudgingly conceded in the case of controversial treatment. But, otherwise, a second opinion was viewed as unnecessary and restrictive, and likely to impede proper patient care. And if there were to be second opinions, the Royal College took the view that they must come from other doctors.

The view of the Royal College is the one which in essence has prevailed. The draft provisions are, not surprisingly, rather complicated, but the professional emerges as the decision-maker. The giving or withholding of consent has been converted into a technical matter, within the unique competence of the doctor to assess. The observation that to be categorized as mentally ill is to run the risk of being robbed of responsibility and the power of self-determination remains valid. Why is this so important? Simply because, in the dispute over consent, and, to an even greater extent, over definitions, what was at stake was power. Changes in the law which tipped the scales towards the individual's civil liberties and the possibility of outside check or review were seen, and quite rightly so, as challenges to the specialists' power. So they were resisted and resisted successfully. In this respect the progress of the Mental Health (Amendment) Act is reminiscent of that of the law which created the NHS. The Government of the day, in both cases, knew that a price had to be paid for the co-operation of the doctors. They, after all, had to operate the system. In the case of the mentally ill, the price has been the retention of power in crucial areas, the continued medicalization of mental illness.

So, it is against this background that I now turn from analysis to prescription. I offer my proposals on how we should approach mental illness in the future. Admittedly, they have been somewhat overtaken by the new draft law. I offer them nonetheless. Some, at least, of the ideas find an echo in the new law, particularly concerning the creation of a more appropriate system of review for those detained as mentally ill. The rest may serve as arguments for the future. I would concede, at the very outset, that there is some validity in the notion of mental illness. It offers us the opportunity to ascribe the status 'ill' to someone whose thoughts or feelings, mood or behaviour, we judge to be abnormal. In granting this status we can offer relief from responsibility to the person designated ill. We can show him that we are prepared to care for him, and about him, and we can allow those who specialize in treating the mentally ill the opportunity to do so, to the extent that we judge their treatments justified. But I am acutely aware of the normative nature of the status, the difficulty of identifying the norm and the implications it carries in terms of loss of liberty and responsibility. So I would seek to define more carefully the criteria of the status 'mentally ill', to limit the circumstances in which it may be applied and thus, by implication, limit the power of the expert. Obviously, I cannot do more than sketch an outline here. I offer a general framework, aware that some degree of vagueness is inevitable.

There would be three classes of person to whom the status

'mentally ill' could be applied. The first class would consist of those who by their conduct, as well as their thinking, become dangerous to others. It would not be enough merely to entertain thoughts which, if carried out, would be dangerous. There would have to be some positive conduct, some action, which posed a threat to the community. In other words, there would have to be conduct which amounted to a violation of the criminal law. Care would then have to be taken to separate the criminal, who ought to be blamed and take moral responsibility, from the person who ought not to be blamed. Given that this is ultimately a moral and social decision, I see no reason why it should not be made by a committee of lay people or a jury. It is not a matter of expertise, since there are no experts possessed of greater insights into what our moral values ought to be than the rest of us. This, I submit, was the approach adopted in the trial of Peter Sutcliffe in 1981. He murdered some eleven women, nine of whom were prostitutes. His defence, which was rejected, was that he was acting on some visitation from God, who appeared to him as he went about his work as a gravedigger. If the person was not to be blamed, yet the danger was sufficiently great, I would condone the compulsory detention of such a person. If he were detained, there would have to be a tribunal or committee, established by law, which would periodically review whether his detention was justified. If it was not, he would, of course, be released. Such a committee or tribunal would, once again, consist of lay people, though, of course, it would hear the views of those claiming expertise. And, of course, the detained person would have all the rights appropriate to someone detained against his will, including an opportunity to appeal and access to an adviser, whether lawyer or layman.

The second class of persons would consist of those who requested help. They would be the unhappy, the depressed, the anguished, those who found the stress of life difficult to bear. It would be for such a person to ask for help; help must not be forced upon him. And, if he chooses to diagnose himself, or let himself be diagnosed, as mentally ill, in that he chooses to consult those who specialize in mental health, then so be it. The usual range of services would be made available to him. There would be no case for admitting such a person to hospital unless he sought or accepted it. Is there not a risk, it may be asked, that some may choose to join this second class, so as to opt out and become free-loaders, living off the State? The answer must be that, if a person chooses to live among us but to look to the State for financial support, beyond free advice and appropriate treatment, he would have to satisfy a panel of lay people that he was unable to provide for himself. In making its decision, the evidence and recommendation of those in whose care he had placed himself, would, of course, be before the panel. But the risk of someone opting to free-load by living in a mental hospital is slim enough not to cause us great concern!

The third and final class would consist of those who ought to be helped, as they appear helpless. This is, of course, a wide and potentially unmanageable category. It looks, I admit, not unlike the woolly sort of categorization I have previously been criticizing. But it need not be. It would differ in that legislation would have to be drafted which was far more carefully and narrowly drawn than the present law. It would differ in that helplessness would be specifically related not to bogus diseases or disorders but to demonstrable facts, which would have to be proved. Such facts would be a person's inability to perform the basic tasks of life, such as procuring food or practising hygiene or finding lodging. It would differ in that provision would be made for distinguishing between the odd, the eccentric or the apparently foolhardy, and the helpless, warranting help. The distinction would turn on choice. If the person chose his way of life and did not request help, then so be it. Some may argue, of course, that the person may have chosen, but his choice was the product of confusion. This is where we came in, where caring becomes controlling, where our values as to how life should be lived are converted into normative propositions as to how others should live. If there is no evidence of choice, no indication that the state in which the person finds himself is the product of his will, then he would warrant help, if otherwise he could not sustain himself.

Some may say this makes no allowance for the person who finds himself in difficulties, not out of choice but out of circumstances which he was powerless to control. I would merely remind them that we are asking here whether such a person should be regarded as mentally ill. I am suggesting he should not be. I am emphatically not suggesting he should be abandoned. But it is the job of others — whether through social services or informally in the community — to cater to his needs, and if possible to restore his dignity. To push him into the embrace of mental illness would not only achieve the opposite, it would also violate the central premise of my whole argument.

By definition, membership of this class would warrant something being done to the helpless person, paternalistic action, without his consent. It would involve compulsion and possibly detention. So provision would have to be made for a formal hearing, before any decision to impose help is made, except in the rare emergency case. Also, provision would be made for periodic review of the detention, so that no one could be forgotten, lost for ever in the back wards. It would differ from the existing situation in that I can see no reason why such decisions should be taken by those claiming expertise. Given the fact that liberty is involved, as well as a sense of caring, it is appropriate that lay people, whether as committee or jury, should decide. This would allow us, in effect, to give substance to our claimed respect for the Samaritan over the Levite, while ensuring that the Samaritan does not become a Zealot or a Pharisee.

You will have noticed that in identifying these three categories I have not referred to the various disease categories at present used, or listed in the law. As I have said, I, like many, have no faith in the validity of these disease labels, whether it be schizophrenia, psychopathy or personality disorder. Under the scheme I propose, only those who come within the three classes I have outlined would be susceptible to being described as mentally ill. If, thereafter, those who treat them wish to ascribe such labels, then so be it. Nor have I referred to those people who may by their conduct represent a danger to themselves rather than to others. I take the view that if freedom and responsibility are to mean anything people must be left to choose to destroy themselves. Otherwise you undermine their sense of responsibility. You categorize them as mentally ill and thereby medicalize them. Perhaps you prevent them from killing themselves on this occasion, but only at a price, to all of us, in terms of the inroads made into the notion of self-determination, and, at a price to them, in terms of how they perceive themselves and their sense of responsibility for themselves in the future.

I am not, of course, arguing for a moment that potential suicides or self-mutilators be ignored. I am merely suggesting they should not be categorized as mentally ill. I would be the first to advocate the creation of social agencies, offering help and support, public or private. A wonderful example of the latter is the Samaritans. But the key to the Samaritans is that the individual has to lift the telephone himself, and, once he calls, he is not classified as mentally ill. Both of these are crucial in the scheme of things I contemplate. I do not suggest, either, that we should abandon the anguished or unhappy, and leave them without care. But, support and care are not uniquely within the gift of those who concern themselves, as professionals, with mental illness. A principal concern of mine is that by medicalizing our response to certain behaviour, we have persuaded ourselves that care is a matter of expertise, which we non-professionals do not have, so that, with a clear conscience, we can wash our hands of the need to care. This can only be regretted. It lessens us as humans.

It only remains to remind you that what I said as regards other illnesses is equally true here. We must redirect our energies and resources towards identifying, and then preventing, the factors which bring about the ills I have described. In mental illness, prevention may go to the root of our culture. This shows us the dimensions of the task. It need not deflect us.

I began by asking you about George, Bill and Tom. You remember George plans to commit suicide, Bill feels hounded by the Inland Revenue, Tom preaches race hatred. They pose problems for us. We can resort to medicine and the arcane skills of those who practise mental health care. But what price do we pay if we do so?

6 'Let's kill all the lawyers'

I have chosen to take as the topic of my sixth chapter* the doctrine of consumerism. Consumerism is a form of social engineering. In the hands of government, administrative agencies, courts, and private interest groups, it can be made to serve the perceived needs of the day, to protect and promote the interests of the consumer. Ordinarily, when we think of consumerism, we think of a movement concerned with the market-place, the buying and selling of goods, making sure that the buyer does not get a pig in a poke or is not taken advantage of in ways which offend current notions of fairness.

The rhetoric of consumerism is couched in terms of consumers' rights. I am not sure that this is helpful. Appeals to rights always strike me as attempts to translate into something more substantial and worthy of respect what are, in effect, merely claims or intuitions. Consumerism is better understood as being concerned with protecting what are judged, at the time, to be the legitimate interests of the consumer, in the face of the greater power of others to hurt or injure or exploit him or to undermine his power of self-determination and responsibility for his own destiny. The aim is for a better balance of power, in the light of prevailing values.

Of course, consumerism is not limited to the market-place. It is just as concerned with the supply of services as with goods. The consumer merely becomes the client, or patient, or whatever, rather than the shopper. For example, the Royal Commission on Legal Services, whose Report appeared in 1979, was set up specifically to consider the extent to which the legal profession was meeting the needs of the community. The way in which medicine is practised and organized is, therefore, equally grist for the mill of consumerism. What does consumerism have to offer in the context of the practice of medicine?

*There are six Reith Lectures and I chose Consumerism as the final one since it seemed to offer a suitable finale in the light of the previous five. Chapter 7 which follows was added subsequent to the presentation of the Lectures.

You will recall that throughout my analysis of medicine I have repeatedly urged on you the need to reshape medicine so that it may better serve our needs. I have also stressed the need for us, as ordinary people, to reclaim some of the power we have chosen to surrender to medicine and medicine men. Does consumerism offer a means of reshaping medicine? Does consumerism offer a means to redress this imbalance of power? It is my contention that consumerism has much to offer. I do not present it as a panacea, nor as the only means available. Clearly, it is one approach among several. But, to me it has great potential. It is a trite observation that only if we are informed can we make responsible choices. One of the great values of consumerism is that intrinsic in it is a commitment to the dissemination of information and an invitation to the education of self and others.

There are, perhaps, three principal areas on which the attention of those advancing the claims of the consumer may focus. The first is the promotion of health. Obviously, consumerism here is very wide-ranging. It can take such forms as lobbying against cigarette advertising, seeking to ensure that cars are designed safely through the passage of appropriate safety legislation, holding inquiries into the safety of nuclear power installations, or regulating the additives which appear in our food. For the most part, action on behalf of the consumer falls to be taken by the Government, since in the promotion of health or prevention of illness all of us are consumers. Equally, as we have seen, it is the Government, national and local, which provides such services for preventive care and the promotion of health as health visitors or health education officers. Part of the strategy I have proposed for the improvement of our health services obviously includes pressure on the Government, by the consumer, for the continued improvement of such services.

Occasionally, individuals, or groups, have acted as champions of certain sections of the community, or of all of us. The various organizations concerned with the elderly or the poor or with handicapped children serve as good examples. By and large, they pursue their goals through the political processes: by lobbying, by producing reports, by promoting legislation. There is no great tradition in this country of using the courts to this end. In the United States, on the other hand, the courts have been most active in advancing the consumer's interest. You will recall that it was Ralph Nader who showed the way, with his spectacular success against General Motors on behalf of the users of cars, described in his book *Unsafe at Any Speed*.

One recent attempt in England was the lawsuit brought in 1979 against several oil companies on behalf of some children living in Birmingham. The allegation was that the lead in petrol, which escaped into the atmosphere through car exhausts, had damaged the health of the children involved, who lived near an area notorious for the volume of traffic and the traffic congestion. The suit was lost, in the face of immense problems of evidence and proof.

It may be that the courts in the United Kingdom are unsuited to engage in this kind of wide-ranging social engineering, and that Parliament is the better place to resolve such problems. But I reach this conclusion not without regret, since, of course, parliamentary time is not as readily given over to the consideration of these issues as is perhaps necessary, given their importance. And, in the commerce of political compromise, concern for the promotion of the health of the community, through measures which rub against established interests and will show no immediate reward, becomes so much small change. It would be a salutary development for all of us if more were willing to take their claims before the courts. Our courts, although traditionally conservative and slow to move, have on occasions shown great willingness to innovate, if the cause can be shown to be just. Indeed, it was the courts who were first to champion the cause of the ordinary consumer in the market-place. Admittedly, for a variety of reasons, courts in the United Kingdom perceive their role quite differently from that adopted by many courts in the United States. Nonetheless, they have been persuaded to venture where others hesitated, and could be persuaded again. I do not suggest that resort to the courts should be the only, or even the principal, means of securing the interests of consumers anxious to promote better health. I do say, however, that it offers another possible opportunity to those whose plea for a shift in the balance of power has met with rejection elsewhere. Indeed, I am fortified in this view by, for example, the test cases brought over the past two or three years by Mind on behalf of the mentally ill. Successful suits have been brought before both the English and Scottish courts and the European Court of Human Rights, when all other forms of action had proved ineffective. The cases have not only had a considerable impact on the treatment of the mentally ill, but also served as an impetus for some of the changes in the law now presaged by the Mental Health (Amendment) Act.

The second area in which consumerism may have some impact is that of medical research. Developments in the medical sciences seem to overtake us at present with such rapidity that new techniques, new medicines, new procedures, have already been adopted into medical practice before we have had any opportunity to subject them to anything approaching careful or measured consideration, far less reach any judgement. We are simply overtaken by the fact that, for example, genetic screening for a whole host of factors is now being engaged in, or by the fact that coronary-bypass surgery or heart-transplant surgery or genetic engineering are not just possibilities but realities. We, the ordinary citizens, have to all intents and purposes been overtaken, overwhelmed by such developments. We have been presented with a series of *faits accomplis*. It is not a question of whether such and such research ought to continue, or be put to practical application. It has become a matter of how we adapt to this development. The medical scientist and technologist have won the day.

Of course, none of the developments I have mentioned, and there are countless others, is free of problems, both practical and ethical. Yet we, the consumers, are rarely heard. But it is we who are affected by these developments, whether as patients or as members of the community, the physical safety or moral integrity of which is challenged. And, if any of us should be bold, or naive, enough to raise his voice and suggest we wait a moment before opening this particular Pandora's box, the scientific establishment reacts with wounded indignation. 'How dare you challenge the right to pursue knowledge, conduct research and introduce technical innovation?' There is that word 'right' again. The flag of Galileo is waved in your face, as code words such as 'censorship' or 'standing in the way of progress' are hurled.

It seems to me that this is a very unsatisfactory state of affairs. I do not need to dwell long on the researcher's arguments, since I find them nonsensical. There has never been a time when we valued the pursuit of knowledge over all things, and this is as true in medicine as elsewhere. Let someone inject an unwanted baby with some agent, known to be toxic, but the precise effects of which are unknown, just to see what happens. He may want to know. He may even feel he has a right to know. But if he makes it as far as the jail in one piece he will certainly have a long time to ponder on the limits of this so-called right.

Clearly, we as consumers may properly assert that the values by which we wish to live simply make doing some things, or introducing some procedures, wrong. But, as I say, by and large, this process of evaluation has gone by the board. One of the principal reasons is ignorance. We do not know, or find it hard to discover, what is happening. There is no conspiracy against us. It is merely that the more technical the exercise, the more it is presumed that it is a matter for technicians to decide upon. This is true as far as the observation whether, for example, a frog which has been the object of an experiment has grown another leg. It is self-evidently not true as regards the more fundamental question, whether the researcher ought to be involved in making frogs with five legs.

There are, of course, circumstances in which reviews are undertaken of the propriety of medical scientific research or the introduction of new procedures. But, with few exceptions, such exercises are fatally flawed. Such committees of review usually consist wholly, or largely, of medical scientists themselves. Take, for example, the committee in the United Kingdom which considered in 1976 the profoundly important question of when someone shall be judged to be dead, a problem created by the development of intensive care techniques and life-support machinery. The Committee, which published its Code of Practice in the *British Medical Journal* of 13 November 1976, consisted, with two exceptions, of physicians and surgeons, some of whom were specialists in transplantation surgery. I offer no criticism of the Code of Practice, nor of the members of the committee. But the association of the Code with transplantation persuades some to reflect whether it may tend to sacrifice the interests of the moribund patient in favour of those of a potential beneficiary of his organs. My view is that the association is unfortunate, but does not, in the event, invalidate the Code. But why were there so few non-medical members, representatives of the rest of us who are not doctors, but who do not need to be to hold a view on the issue of death? Equally, in 1979 a working party set up by the DHSS published its report on antenatal screening to detect the condition called spina bifida. The technical complexities are considerable. But so too are the financial, and therefore political, the ethical and hence the moral implications. Yet the working party consisted of twelve doctors and two nurses.

It seems clear to me that better machinery must be established to monitor the progress of medical research and the introduction of new practices and procedures. We are entitled to ask, for example, what such an institutional mechanism, a review committee, for example, with a membership drawn from a cross-section of the community, would have recommended when faced with the proposal to re-start heart-transplant operations in England in 1979. In the event, two centres began to perform these operations again, without apparent reference to the views of the larger community as to the propriety of doing so, whether ethically, socially, or in terms of the proper allocation of scarce resources. The Department of Health had refused to finance heart-transplant operations several years previously, but private financial support was made available.

It is fair to say that some progress along the lines I advocate has recently been made. The British Medical Association has invited non-doctors to participate in its deliberations on ethics in research. Furthermore, the Committees set up in 1982 by the Royal College of Obstetricians and Gynaecologists and by the DHSS, to consider research into reproduction, with particular reference to *in vitro* fertilization, both contain a liberal sprinkling of members who are neither doctors nor research scientists. Indeed, the DHSS Committee will be chaired by a distinguished moral philosopher, Mary Warnock. The drawback of such groups is, as I have said already, that they tend to be *ad hoc* and to disperse once their immediate task is done. You will recall that I have already discussed in some detail the formal mechanism I would favour for the consideration and resolution of problems of medical ethics. I suggested that an appropriately constituted Permanent Standing Advisory Committee be appointed with a permanent secretariat. As an alternative to the present unsatisfactory state of affairs, there is no reason why such a Committee's brief should not extend to monitoring medical research, since many of the problems are ethical in nature.

As an alternative, a committee or group with more specific terms of reference could be set up. There is already in operation a good example of the sort of institutional arrangement I envisage, in the committee created to oversee developments in genetic engineering. It is called the Genetic Manipulation Advisory Group and was created in 1976. The membership naturally includes those conversant with the technical details. But it also includes, for example, trades unionists, scientists from other disciplines and others drawn from a variety of backgrounds. To those who protest at this intrusion into the field of medical scientific research, the reply must be that only in this way can we, the consumers, for whom new procedures and practices are intended, have our voice heard before it is too late.

In the United States, developments have gone much further, particularly at the instigation of the Federal Government. The Department of Health and Human Resources has created a series of ethics committees charged with the task of overseeing research and development, and we have already taken note of the President's Commission on (among other things) Biomedical and Behavioral Research. There is, of course, the inevitable danger of bureaucratization, as well as the objections already noted. By and large, however, I feel we have much to learn from how this aspect of consumerism has developed in the United States.

Let me now, for a moment, refer back to research in reproductive medicine and, particularly, *in vitro* fertilization. Obviously, it is simply pointless to argue, although some do, that *in vitro* fertilization (IVF), as a technique for overcoming infertility in couples, should be stopped because it poses too many ethical problems. The fact is that it is with us and cannot be stopped. This is not to say, however, that it should not be controlled in some appropriate way, nor that some practices associated with it should not be prevented, if it were thought right. There is no doubt a pressing need to lay down and enforce some guidelines in this area. There is something of the frontiersman about some of the researchers; on their own, taming nature, making the law as they go, building a future our children can inherit. But others are sufficiently concerned about some aspects of the research to propose a moratorium while we all take stock, while others call for a ban on them.

I want here to consider some of the more urgent problems which arise. Before I go any further, however, I want to draw your attention to a point which pervades all thinking about IVF and thus has as much relevance to the researcher as to the doctor dealing with the infertile couple, but is often overlooked. This is the idea that there exists a right to have a family. This assumption or assertion needs close analysis. For if it is allowed to pass without comment, the researcher and doctor involved in IVF, as in other areas of reproductive medicine, can rationalize their conduct and resist the scrutiny of others by arguing that all they are doing is 'helping' a mother or a couple to satisfy their right to have a family. This casting of the researcher or doctor in the role of helper serves to play down, or even dismiss, the ethical complexities of the procedures they are engaged in. It allows them, in effect, to wash their hands of the difficult moral problems since, after all, they are merely agents helping others attain their rights and, therefore, must be on the side of good whatever they do.

Admittedly, the European Convention of Human Rights asserts, in Article 12, the right to marry and 'found a family'. But the question remains of whether limits exist or ought to exist to the exercise of this right. It may not be right morally to seek to gratify the desire of someone for a child in *all* circumstances. And notice here that we are talking of gratifying a desire for pregnancy which, otherwise, cannot be realized; we are not talking of how to respond once a woman has become pregnant. It is possible to think of categories of claimant who are obviously acceptable — for example, the stable, loving, happily married couple. But what of the 99 per cent of other couples! It must be true that there are claimants whose desire to found a family ought not to be readily satisfied. The point is that, indeed, it is for the researcher and doctor and others to help, but it is essential to ask whom they should help, what are the relevant guiding principles, and who decides on them. Clearly, deciding who should benefit from services designed to facilitate the creation of a family is no simple exercise. It has about it an aura of eugenics which is undeniable and must be confronted. The fact is, of course, that such decisions are already being made, idiosyncratically, by individual doctors and parents. My contention is that they ought to be made by reference to principles set by all of us. For I take the view that when we are considering the circumstances under which a family ought to be brought into being, we all have a right to be heard. What is involved is too serious to be merely a matter of private treaty between doctor and patient. Some may well argue that this is unnecessary, or intrusive, or even invasive of the rights of couples to satisfy their desire for a family. After all, it is said, families are created in the most haphazard and unsupervised and, perhaps, even undesirable fashion as a consequence of natural reproduction. My reply would be that, while this may be true, it does not mean we ought to replicate nature when we have the ability to do otherwise.

Whatever view is taken on these points it seems to me that as a matter of great urgency there is a need to answer the questions posed by practices associated with IVF in an authoritative and morally respectable way.

Of the more urgent problems, the first I want to touch on is that of the surrogate mother. This is the woman who agrees to carry in her womb to term the fertilized egg of a couple. She may do so because the woman who supplies the egg cannot bear her own child or for less worthwhile motives. On the basis of present information, my response to this is draconian. I would outlaw the practice. I would make it a crime for a woman to do this, or for others to aid and abet her. I must, of course, offer good reasons for so drastic a solution. I would remind you that the basis for all regulation in this area of medicine must be what is in the best interests of the child. It seems to me that the confusions and ambiguities which would arise from what would appear to be two natural mothers, and possible competition between them, make it hard to argue that it would be in the child's best interests to be born into such circumstances. It may well be that children born in normal circumstances face similar sorts of problems when they are adopted, or one parent remarries, but the situation is by no means the same, and the traditional difficulties encountered by children in such contexts serve as a good ground for avoiding them when it is in our power to do so. A childless couple can, after all, have recourse to adoption to found a family if their desire is so great. To go beyond that, to hire the body of a woman, is to go too far. It is not necessarily right that childlessness should always go remedied, whatever the remedy.

I turn next to the carrying out of experiments or tests on embryos produced as a consequence of IVF. It has become part of the research endeavour of a number of medical scientists to use some embryos at a very early stage of their development from eggs fertilized *in vitro* for the purpose of research. It seems to me that this is morally objectionable. For this reason I would again argue that it be outlawed, since no other form of control or exhortation is likely to prevent or control it. To leave regulation to professional self-discipline or individual consciousness would not be enough. Nor would it reflect the seriousness with which the State ought to regard the question. The moral objection lies in the fact that what the researcher is doing is facilitating the creation of an entity, with a potential for human life, for the sole purpose of conducting research on it and then letting it die.

To those who argue that this is no more objectionable than abortion, which I would defend as a practice in most circumstances, I would point to the intention of the researcher. In both cases the death of the embryo (or foetus in the case of abortion) is intended. But in the case of research, the intention is to cause the bringing about of life *only for the purpose of research* and with the intention, thereafter, of letting it die. The response could be made, as regards research on embryos produced through IVF, that the intention of the researcher was not to create an embryo only for the purpose of research. Often, a woman who is trying to become pregnant through IVF will be caused to produce several eggs at ovulation. This enables the doctor to implant more than one in the woman's womb, so as to maximize the chances of her becoming pregnant. There may be embryos left over, however, and it is these which may be the objects of experiments. In such a case, the researcher or doctor can argue that he did not create the embryo with a view to experimenting on it, since he did not know whether all attempts to fertilize the eggs he had available would be successful. Furthermore, since the embryo is available and will suffer no pain, he can say that he may, indeed ought to, use the embryo as research material to benefit future children. The answer to this argument must be that he intentionally created more embryos than he would need, since he knew he would not need all, so that he did, in fact, create the embryo for the purpose of research. Alternatively, once he had created the embryo, by not placing it in the womb he had denied it the chance to survive and it is adding to the moral wrong to treat it as a thing to be created, used and then discarded.

To those who argue that any such ban on research would place a major obstacle in the way of those working in the area of IVF and infertility, or in immunology, indeed in the whole field of genetics, I would remind you that there are a number of circumstances in which the need to know must be subordinated to respect for other, more highly prized, values. The cost of knowing in the case of research on the embryo is too high, in terms of the threat it poses to the respect all of us should pay to the uniqueness of the potential for human life, and the spiritual awesomeness of the creation of life. Such creation should not be seen as a mere convenience for gaining ephemeral understanding. My opposition, then, in short, is born of a fundamental distaste for the idea of something with the potential for human life being created for the purpose of, or, having been created, being earmarked for, experiments before being left to die.

The last question I want to consider concerns the storage of embryos. It now is possible to preserve embryos for long periods of time and indeed some researchers have begun to do so, or announced their intention of doing so. Provided that the ultimate donee of the embryo when it is removed from storage is the woman, or the couple, whose fertilized egg it is, I cannot see any greater moral problems than those I have already mentioned as regards IVF in general. But this is subject to the proviso that the storage process does not cause damage to the embryo, and hence the child. This is a most important proviso and one which must be made, if concern for the best interests of the child is to be paramount. The difficulty with such a proviso is, of course, that it cannot be known whether the storage process causes damage unless someone stores an embryo and then implants it and brings it to term. And, by then, the damage, if any, would be done. It must follow that embryo storage is also an unethical enterprise because of the unknown but real risk of harm to embryo and child. If it is wrong, what form should the prohibition against it take? Since I suspect exhortation or informal control again would not be effective, again I conclude that the practice ought to be made illegal.

Because of this conclusion, it is unnecessary to consider as a separate problem the situation in which the stored embryo is implanted into a woman who did not provide the fertilized egg. If it were necessary, I would regard this as akin to the situation of the surrogate mother, thereby warranting the same opposition.

I offer these arguments for consideration. I am sure many would dispute them. The various Committees set up to review these and other matters associated with IVF will reach their conclusions in due course. Then issue can be joined and some policy formed. Though holding the views I have expressed above, I am content to fall in with the approach set out so well in *The Times* editorial of 19 April 1982: ' . . . The issues raised by the rapid technical advances in this field extend far beyond immediate questions of medical practice. They are connected with deep feelings about individual rights and the nature of the family, and fears about the power of science . . . Techniques already developed as part of existing procedures open out . . . bizarre possibilities. Unfertilized and probably fertilized genetic material can be frozen alive for long periods. Fertilized ova can be divided at an early stage of growth to be tested for genetic defects: each divided section could in principle grow into a complete individual, and unlimited numbers of identical twins could in theory be produced in this way. Destroying such material or experimenting on it, or even buying and selling it, raise novel problems of human rights. The law has nothing to say on the question of whose child such an embryo would be if implanted in an unrelated woman. The laws of inheritance and legitimacy were framed without regard to such possibilities. Legislation will be required once consensus is achieved, and a full public inquiry is needed to start the process. If it is put off till some scandal forces the issue, it will be too late: the time is now.'

My third area in which consumerism has a role to play is the much more specific and more important one of the actual day-to-day practice of medicine. This is where consumerism can and should make its greatest impact. In the practice of medicine, the consumer is the patient. His interests, which consumerism seeks to assert, are those of self-determination and the power to participate responsibly in decisions made about his life. The challenge to that power comes from the doctor who, in the exercise of his professional role, threatens to infantilize his patient, to undermine his power of self-determination, to act in a paternalistic manner. Consumerism has a role to play in establishing standards which doctors must meet in their practice, in measuring the doctor's performance in the light of these standards, and in creating means of redress for the patient and sanctions against the doctors, if these standards are breached. And when I refer to standards, I think it is important to note that there are two areas of concern for the consumer. One involves ensuring that the doctor meets the appropriate standards of technical competence, the other that he meets the required ethical standards.

How can consumerism play these various roles I have outlined – setting standards, measuring performance and providing remedies or sanctions? There are several approaches. They are not mutually exclusive. We should consider each of them carefully. If all of them were implemented, it would not only be the patient who would gain. The doctor too would benefit, as would the practice of medicine.

The most obvious approach is professional self-regulation. This is an odd, paternalistic kind of consumerism, in which the professional presumes to be the sympathetic advocate of the consumers' interests. The medical profession already claims to be a self-regulating body, both in matters of technical competence and ethical propriety. The General Medical Council establishes standards and seeks to ensure that they are observed. But the Council is less concerned with competence than with ethics, and less concerned with ethics than with etiquette. The various Royal Colleges, for example of Surgery or Psychiatry or General Practice, also set standards of professional competence which must be reached before the doctor has access to certain appointments.

That this is not enough, particularly in the realm of competence, that more is needed, is recognized, at least tacitly, by the relatively recent establishment in a number of hospitals of a mechanism called

162

'peer review'. This involves a regular review and critical examination of, for example, the treatment programmes adopted by each member of the staff. Another method of self-regulation is the formal establishment of what is called 'professional audit'. As its name suggests, doctors review and evaluate their own and their colleagues' clinical methods, with a view to improvement. This is an area where there is much to be learned from experience in the United States. In 1972 Professional Standards Review Organizations (PSROs) were introduced by the Federal Government to monitor the performance of doctors working within the federally funded Medicare and Medicaid programmes, providing care for the poor and elderly. Despite the initial hostility to them and the fact that they are limited to these programmes, there is little doubt that the PSROs are of some, albeit limited, value in safeguarding the interests of the consumer.

But audits, as yet, are relatively uncommon. One reason is that there are no clear guides as to the standards to be applied. The conclusion of the Royal Commission on the NHS was that it was 'not convinced that the profession generally regards the introduction of audit or peer review of standards of care and treatment with a proper sense of urgency'.

This is something of an understatement. Adopting what *The Times* of 12 July 1980 described as a 'strongly defensive attitude' at the 1980 annual representative meeting, the British Medical Association rejected the notion of introducing any form of imposed medical audit. It was, according to one member, 'unnecessary, undesirable, and, in some ways, offensive'.

Finally, randomized controlled trials (RCTs), so vigorously endorsed by Professor Cochrane in his seminal book, *Effectiveness and Efficiency: Random Reflections on Health Services*, have, in his words, been 'much neglected'. Cochrane's thesis is that the effectiveness and usefulness of many forms of treatment have never been clearly demonstrated and that RCTs are of primary importance in safeguarding the interests of patients. The Royal Commission concluded that 'there seems little doubt that the more widespread use of RCTs could eliminate procedures whose benefits are at present accepted simply because they have never been systematically challenged'. Yet, for one reason or another, RCTs continue to be ignored.

Of course, even when it exists, professional self-regulation is always open to the criticism that it is not sufficiently energetic, that ranks will be closed to protect a fellow member, rather than opened to admit the questioning outsider. Certainly, the medical profession can never be expected to become the champion of the consumers' cause. When measures as innocuous as self-audit are met with hostile rejection, it is clear that other approaches on behalf of the consumer are called for. The profession is not going to help. Standards will have to be set and measured by others. The principle of outside scrutiny, a key feature of consumerism, seems inevitable.

One solution could be for Parliament to pass legislation on the consumer's behalf. Certainly, as regards the buying and selling of goods, Parliament has been most active. But in the context of the practice of medicine it has avoided laying down, through legislation, all but the most general guidelines within which medicine is to be practised. What Parliament has preferred to do is either leave matters to the profession or establish independent agencies, charged with advancing the interests of the patient, for example Community Health Councils or the Health Services Commissioner (the Ombudsman). The effectiveness of these agencies depends on their having terms of reference which enable them to do their jobs successfully, and on their receiving appropriate co-operation from the medical profession. The attitude of doctors is crucial. If doctors perceive the agencies as adversaries, rather than partners in the pursuit of a high quality of medical care and service, then the effectiveness of the agencies is much reduced. Sadly, once again, the attitude of many doctors is one of hostility. More than most other groups, doctors have a highly developed sense of territoriality. Having fought hard to gain their professional independence, it is, of course, almost inevitable that they should seek to guard their achievement. Regrettably, many doctors, especially those who act as spokesmen of medical opinion, seem to translate this natural tendency into an uncritical rejection of even the slightest move towards consumerism. Furthermore, the terms of reference of these agencies are an additional barrier to their successful advocacy of the consumers' interests. It is not clear whether it is within their brief to monitor competence, or ethical propriety, or simply bad communication and unprofessionalism.

Take, for example, the Community Health Councils, established in 1974. Members are appointed by local authorities, voluntary organizations and the Regional Health Authority. These councils were conceived of as bodies to represent the views of the consumer, according to the 1972 Government White Paper. They were to monitor services and inform the public. But, as the Royal Commission on the NHS points out, the Councils are widely criticized by doctors as being a waste of money in hard times. As the East Hertfordshire Community Health Council submitted, in its evidence to the Royal Commission, 'the system is loaded against the Community Health Council. It has little money, few staff and no sanctions, save those of public opinion.' The British Medical Association, at their 1980 annual meeting, recommended their abolition, complaining that they were 'interfering in matters that did not concern them'. They were described as 'unhelpful and disruptive'. The attitude of doctors is one of, 'Hands off. We doctors know what is best. Just leave it to us.' Indeed, the present Government even, for some time, toyed with the idea of abolishing the whole system of Community Health Councils. In this climate, it cannot be a surprise that they have not produced the kind of consumer service that might have been expected of them.

Other mechanisms established by government attract the same opprobrium, and have equally been less effective than may be necessary in advancing patients' interests. Take the matter of complaints and the ways in which they are dealt with. An established complaints procedure does exist as regards GPs. But the procedures are altogether less than satisfactory. All complaints must be made in writing to the appropriate body within eight weeks of the event complained of. The system is excessively formal, takes too much time, is too complicated, and involves complaining to the very body which administers the GP service. There was no formal statutory complaints system, as regards medical care in hospitals, until one was introduced, as we shall see, on a trial basis in September 1981. The Parliamentary Select Committee on the Ombudsman, in its 1977 Report, severely criticized the existing system for dealing with complaints in hospitals. The procedures were condemned as complicated, fragmented and slow. Complainants were, the Committee said, often left dissatisfied, particularly when a clinical element was involved in the case.

Clearly, if it is thought desirable that complaints should be dealt with administratively within the Health Service, the system was in need of a thoroughgoing reform. One suggestion for reform has been to extend the powers of the Ombudsman. At present, he has a very limited jurisdiction. The great majority of complaints he receives, about 80 per cent, are held to be outside his jurisdiction. One particular limit is that he may not inquire into matters involving a doctor's clinical judgement, a phrase which is, of course, delightfully vague. So the suggestion has been made that his jurisdiction should be extended, by giving him the power to inquire into clinical matters. The Parliamentary Select Committee recommended this in 1977, as did the Royal Commission on the NHS. Predictably, the BMA at their 1980 meeting, rejected the idea unanimously.

What happened instead was that the hospital doctors came up with their own complaints procedure, in matters of clinical judgement. Realizing which way the wind was blowing they decided to get their ideas in first before anyone else had different ideas. Perhaps I can take a moment to look at this procedure in greater detail, as it represents the latest development in medical political thinking in the hospital sector. Published in November 1980, the procedure was accepted by the Government on 18 April, and implemented on 1 September 1981. Quite frankly, the hospital doctors have pulled off a considerable political coup. For the complaints procedure is hardly what you would call a consumer's charter. In his introduction to it, David Bolt, Chairman of the BMA's Central Committee for Hospital Medical Services and a consultant surgeon, wrote, in the *British Medical Journal* of 22 November 1980, how 'strongly opposed' the 'entire medical profession' was to the idea of extending the role of the Ombudsman. The Secretary of State at the DHSS, 'wishing', he went on, 'to avoid the problems which would result from the imposition of the authority of the Ombudsman by legislation without prior agreement, has made clear his concern that the profession should find a solution to this difficulty.' Note that Mr Bolt uses the words 'would result', not could, or may, result.

The solution which the hospital doctors found was a procedure which entails three possible stages. The first stage is designed to solve complaints of a 'less serious nature' by direct communication between doctor and patient. If the patient is not content with this, we move to stage two. This contemplates either further talk between the two of them, after the doctor has had an opportunity to consult colleagues, or, if this gets nowhere, the chance to move to stage three. At stage three, two independent consultants will consider the complaint. They may decide all is well and seek to persuade the patient of this, or, if they decide otherwise, they will explain to the complainant, 'as far as appropriate, how it was hoped to overcome the problems which had been identified'. Or, as Mr Bolt put it, '*assure* the complainant that adequate steps *had been taken* to prevent a similar occurrence in the future' (my emphasis). If, at stage three, it appears that the case is 'exceptional', the two consultants should recommend 'that the complaint would be best pursued by alternative means'. This presumably refers to the possibility of legal action. The main thrust, as Mr Bolt candidly writes, is, first, to deal with complaints 'by direct discussion with the complainant, *without other interference*' (my emphasis). Where this fails, 'the great majority of complaints would be dealt with by colleagues, *keeping the matter within the profession*, and seeking expert help in *reassuring* the complainant that all proper steps *had been taken and appropriate skill exercised*' (my emphasis). And there is more in this vein. Take, for example, Mr Bolt's advice that 'written communication with the regional medical officer [required for stage two] would be confined to the minimum required to inform him of the action taken, so as to minimize material which could be subpoenaed'. This gives a new, and perhaps more realistic, meaning to the words 'defensive medicine'. I find myself out of sympathy with this approach.

The picture is depressing. It may be that the interests of patients could be advanced through appropriate administrative agencies, but it is clear that the present arrangements are wholly inadequate to the task. Successive governments have been prepared to do little or nothing, until something awful attracts the attention of the press, when they deplore it as if it were not their responsibility. As the Royal Commission complained, 'It is neither just nor efficient to allow one scandal after another to erupt, to institute an inquiry and then to pillory those who have drifted into the often neglected services.' For the most part, it has been left to private charitable organizations, such as Mind or Age Concern, to champion the patients' cause. The medical profession seems bent on an unyielding policy of hostility to what it perceives as attacks on its professional integrity. For example, the Royal College of General Practitioners found that two-thirds of the GPs in the study it conducted, and these were GPs training young doctors, were unaware of patient participation groups in family practices. 'Only "That's Life" freaks*, hypochondriacs, committee types and bored housewives would be likely to join,' was the view expressed. In fact, the first group was established in 1963 and all of them were begun by doctors.

*'That's Life' is a popular television programme concerned with consumerism.

The opposition of the medical profession seems total. As the inept *Handbook of Medical Ethics*, revised most recently in 1980 by the BMA, declares, 'The ideal personal doctor service . . . can exist only when the limits to it set by the state are so wide that in day-to-day practice there are no practical constraints.' This sort of stubborn intransigence is unjustified, not only from an ethical point of view, particularly in a profession which claims that its relationship with patients rests on trust, and then demands to be trusted. It is also clearly out of line with the political tenor of the day. Consumerism is with us. The doctor has the choices only of accepting it willingly and co-operating, or accepting it unwillingly.

The most contentious approach to furthering the interests of patients in matters of technical competence, and sometimes of ethical propriety, when law and ethics overlap, is private litigation, suing doctors or hospital administrations or others involved in medical care. Even the mention of this raises the hackles of the medical profession. You can hear the protests forming. Nothing could be more damaging to the future of medical care than the suggestion that patients sue their doctors. But, if you accept that the power and freedom of the patient are in need of assertion, or protection, you have already seen that existing ways of achieving this are less than outstanding successes. Self-help, in the form of litigation, may then warrant careful consideration. My view is that it does have some role to play, though rather a limited one, in establishing standards of practice and ensuring that they are met.

Of course, mention litigation — suing doctors — and most people will immediately think of the United States. Indeed, one of the problems which bedevils any examination of this aspect of consumerism is the passion it engenders. And this passion is largely the product of unthinking and misinformed allusions to conditions in the United States. So we have to tread slowly and carefully. We have to navigate in an area in which a poster such as 'Support a lawyer. Send your child to medical school' is one of the milder forms of comment from the medical profession.

Let us consider some examples of consumerism through litigation, in the context of medical practice. The first example is a highly charged topic, known in the United States as the doctrine of informed consent. This has not gained much ground yet in the United Kingdom. It is the product wholly of courts, of case law not statute law, and represents the courts' response to what is seen as an unmet need.

It represents an attempt to give greater emphasis to the well recognized ethical principle of respecting autonomy through informed consent, by translating it into law, so signifying the importance society attaches to it. The legal doctrine of informed consent, simply stated, has it that a doctor has an obligation in law to obtain the consent of his patient before embarking on any procedure. But it goes much further than that, as can be seen, for instance, in the famous California case of *Cobbs* v. *Grant,* decided in 1972. For it also requires doctors to advise their patients of all material risks involved in the proposed procedure, so that the patient may make an informed decision on what course to take. Clearly, this is a classic exercise in consumerism. The patient is the consumer, utterly dependent on the professional, and therefore given a right of redress if he is subsequently harmed. As a doctrine, informed consent flies the flag of self-determination against the otherwise ever-present paternalism of the doctor.

For years, doctors have responded to patients' questions with answers such as 'Don't worry about that' or 'Leave it to me'. They have even persuaded patients to agree that the doctor, in performing any procedure or operation, may do whatever he thinks is necessary. For example, women have had breasts removed without being consulted, after biopsy has shown the presence of a tumour, or have undergone a regime of hormone treatment ignorant of and therefore unprepared for some of the effects it has produced. Consumerism is designed, here, to protect the interests of the consumer, the patient, by requiring that the final decision as to what shall be done to his body rests with him and not with the doctor. And, of course, it has been reviled by a large sector of the medical profession, as interfering in, and thereby damaging, the delicate relationship between doctor and patient. As I have said, it is a legal doctrine far more highly developed in the United States. Doctors and lawyers in the United Kingdom seem to delight in ridiculing this development in the United States, and preaching strongly against any movement towards it. The ridicule is, in my view, unwarranted and born largely of the sort of chauvinistic and lofty ignorance which the English have developed into a higher art form. Of course, there are examples in the United States of unjustified litigation, of unscrupulous patients and lawyers and excessive awards of damages. But these are the exception. Indeed, they are even more exceptional, if you omit reference to just two States, California and New York. And it is important to note that

English law has recently taken a tentative step towards embracing the doctrine more fully. This is clear from the case of *Chatterton* v. *Gerson*, decided in 1981. In this case the court was prepared to state that, as a matter of law, a doctor was under a duty to explain what he intended to do and its implications. I say that the court has made a tentative step, because it only requires the doctor to act as a reasonable doctor would be expected to act, rather than as a reasonable patient might be entitled to expect him to act. Thus, the particular details of this duty, what level of explanation is appropriate and what exceptions may exist, still await clarification. But the principle has been asserted, or reasserted. The position of the consumer, the patient, has been made a little clearer and a little stronger.

There is little doubt that consumerism, in the form of the doctrine of informed consent, promises to transform the doctor–patient relationship. It reasserts the notion that the patient is a partner in any enterprise concerning his health and cannot be a partner if he is kept in ignorance. Just as important, the patient owes it to himself to take responsibility for himself, thereby redressing the balance of power between him and the doctor. That the doctrine had to be developed by courts may be unfortunate to some, but it had to be developed by them simply because there was no other agency willing or able to enforce a proper observance of the ethical principle, which, while universally acknowledged, was systematically ignored. The hope exists that now that the courts have shown their willingness to enforce it, the regrettable need for recourse to the courts will be much reduced.

The legal doctrine of informed consent as it is now operated in the United States has undergone a considerable development from its original premise. Here is where misunderstanding comes in. The courts have expanded the doctrine. Patients suffering unexpected harm have sued their doctors and been successful, even in circumstances where, in the view of most, the doctors have not been at fault, where they have done all that could have been expected of them. Take the case of an otherwise healthy woman about to undergo an operation for a leg injury, caused by jogging. The surgeon visits her and explains in general terms what the operation involves. He does not mention — who would? — that there have been two reported cases in the literature of complications following this operation. After all, the operation has been performed many hundreds of times. Her operation becomes the third to be followed by complications. She sues her surgeon, claiming she did not consent to the operation because she was not informed. This is what makes doctors furious. The doctor has done all he can, all that anyone would expect, yet the patient, because she now, unexpectedly, has unsightly scars or a limp, is seeking money by suing him.

The explanation is not hard to find. There is no well developed health service, of the kind we in the United Kingdom have, in the United States. The old and very poor get health care, of a sort, free of charge. The rest depend on their insurance cover, which often is inadequate, or on savings. Other social welfare benefits of the range provided here are also less available. Thus, if someone suffers harm unexpectedly, he needs money to pay for additional medical care or to meet other costs. With no one else to look to, the best source of money is the insurance carried by the doctor. The patient has made some small contribution to this when he paid his fee to the doctor and, after all, it is not the doctor who will pay, it is his insurer. The doctor will pass on the costs of his insurance premium by spreading them among his patients in the fees he collects. To get this money, however, the patient must sue the doctor and the doctor must be found liable. And, in holding him liable, it appears that the court is saying that he did something wrong, he failed to obtain informed consent. In truth, the court is merely ensuring that some form of social welfare system operates, paid out by insurance and funded from patients' fees. It has to do it by the sleight of hand of judging doctors to be at fault and therefore liable to their patients. Perhaps it would be more honest if the courts said that doctors should be liable regardless of any question of their fault. This is, in fact, the effect of their decisions, even though they are expressed in terms of a failure by the doctor to obtain informed consent. The object of the exercise is, after all, to compensate where compensation is needed, and the doctor's insurance is the best source available. But the American courts have as yet been reluctant to go so far as to endorse openly liability without fault, perhaps for fear that, if they were so honest, the powerful lobby of the medical establishment might persuade the Legislatures to take action to limit by statute the courts' power in this area.

A system of adequate health care, free of charge, and an adequate welfare system would, of course, obviate the need for this form of consumerism, at least as a device for compensating patients who have suffered harm. But in the United States they do not exist in any comprehensive form. Until they do, using the doctor's insurance to pay for patients' needs is as good a solution as any. Clearly, there are numerous disadvantages. As insurance premiums go up to meet claims, so must the doctor's fees go up, so that some would-be patients are priced out of the market. There are some unjustified claims. Doctors are persuaded to practise defensive medicine in the vain hope of avoiding liability. And, finally, some of the openness in the relationship with the patient has been eroded (rather than enhanced), in that doctors have resorted to hiding behind consent forms, carefully, but again, often vainly, drafted by lawyers, instead of talking to their patients. For, ironically, the intervention of the courts was intended to produce, with the best will in the world, a greater dialogue between doctor and patient. It has produced instead a monologue, in which the consent form is made to do the talking.

In the United Kingdom, on the other hand, there is still a social welfare system and free health care, at least for the moment, which can serve as the basic source of funds for patients who complain of harm. So there is obviously less need in the United Kingdom for this form of consumerist litigation, so common in the United States, in which money is the sole objective. But consumerism, in the context of informed consent, is not concerned only with procuring money compensation when harm is suffered. It is concerned as much with establishing the principle of respect for the established legal rights or claims of the patient, which grow out of the ethical principle of informed consent, one of which is his power of self-determination. So it may be that litigation, or the threat of litigation, *is* needed in circumstances in which the protection of this principle is the objective. Furthermore, given the profession's reluctance to discipline its members, litigation could well provide the necessary sanction, or impetus, to ensure that proper standards are observed. I would not regard it as a bad thing if more lawsuits were brought against doctors or hospitals in, for example, cases in which a patient was used as a subject in a clinical trial of a new drug without his knowledge, or in a case in which the full implications of a particular form of treatment were not explained to the patient, or were discussed only with relatives or the patient's spouse. This is the strategy of the test case. It has been used to great effect by, for example, Mind. Practices have been challenged, or the law clarified, on behalf of all the mentally ill, by taking a carefully selected case from which a generalizable rule can emerge. Such actions would, in my view, lead to a healthier respect for the patient's interests and responsibilities than at present seems to exist. And they would tend to ensure that standards of practice were established which met the approval of outsiders, and were adhered to.

An even more widespread form of consumer litigation in the United States is the action for negligence in circumstances other than the failure to obtain informed consent. The patient claims that he has suffered harm because of the failure of the doctor or hospital to behave in a way which could reasonably have been expected of them. Although the number of cases brought each year in the United Kingdom is rising, it is still a very small number, many, many times smaller than the number in the United States. The reasons are complex. There are cultural differences, in that, unlike the Briton, the American is more willing to have recourse to the courts, and less willing to accept what he may see as second best, since he is paying for it. There are differences born of the greater resort to surgery in the United States than in the United Kingdom. Surgery carries greater risk of harm than less invasive forms of therapy, but in the United States it produces higher fees, which doctors have come to regard as their due. Indeed, in more general terms, it is fair to say that doctors in the United States have tended to abandon primary care in favour of high-cost specialities. And with the growth of specialization comes lack of development of any close relationship with the doctor, which is another explanation for a greater willingness to resort to litigation when things go wrong.

But by far the most important difference is that, once again, the patient in the United Kingdom has less incentive to sue, because he has less need of the money which success in the lawsuit would bring. Once again, the British patient needing further care, or disabled in any way, can look initially to the Health Service and social security. His American counterpart can expect less, so must get the money he needs through the informal and expensive social security system of the doctor's insurance. Despite publicity to the contrary, the sums awarded in the United States will not be great. On average, a successful claimant can expect about £7,000 to £15,000 which, given the cost of further health care for example, is not high. So, when the need of the patient is for money compensation for harm suffered, consumerism through the action for negligence fills a need in the United States which is already largely met in the United Kingdom.

But consumerism may have two additional goals. The first is to provide money, when the state system does not provide enough. The second is to ensure that the doctor observes standards which respect the interests of the patient. Can the action for negligence achieve either of these? First, take the case in which a patient is harmed, for whatever reason, and is in need of money to purchase care over and above that available from existing social security sources.

You will recall the case in Birmingham, the case of *Whitehouse* v. *Jordan*.* In December 1979, the Court of Appeal threw out a judgement for £100,000 awarded to a little boy who suffered severe brain damage at birth. Their decision was affirmed by the House of Lords in December 1980. Amid all the trumpeting over the vindication of the doctor, people seemed to lose sight of the realities of the case. This was one of those cases in which a large amount of money was needed to pay for care which was called for, beyond what was forthcoming from the State. The question really before the court was, simply, who should pay. One option was the little boy's parents. This would mean that he would get nothing, as they had no money. It would mean that his mother would struggle on, as she had done for almost eleven long years before the case even reached the House of Lords. Another option was the doctor. The court would have had to decide that the doctor was negligent. Sometimes doctors are incompetent. But this is not often the case. The House of Lords in the Birmingham case decided that the doctor had behaved reasonably and competently. The court could still, however, have decided that he was negligent. But, you say, this sounds contradictory, that the court first decides the doctor has done nothing wrong and then decides he was negligent. It need not be contradictory. It would merely involve redefining the concept of negligence. In common speech, negligence may well still mean carelessness. But its legal meaning need not be the same. Take the words insanity or duress. Their meaning in terms of law is quite different from the meaning they have in common speech.

After all, negligence is merely a legal device. It is flexible. Its meaning is not set in stone for ever. It, like the whole of the law, is dynamic. Just as social circumstances and social needs change, so must the law change and adapt. Negligence is a legal tool doing a job. If the job changes, the tool can be reshaped. It could have given the court the chance to develop the law, so as to give the little boy the money he needed. The court could have decided that, even in the *absence* of fault on the part of the doctor, he *was negligent*, by redefining negligence. This, in the view of many, is what has happened in the United States. Negligence there has lost much of its quality of blame-

*I should mention that it was a namesake, not I, who was counsel for Dr Jordan.

worthiness or fault. Of course, doctors who are found negligent get hopping mad. They have not been negligent, they argue, meaning they have not done anything wrong. They do not understand, because it is not made clear to them, that negligence is no more than a legal device allowing a particular socially desirable conclusion to be arrived at. It has become a convenient device whereby needed money can be channelled to those who have become the casualties of modern medicine.

But why, you ask, do the courts have to talk of negligence at all, since it does inevitably carry that tag of carelessness which harms a doctor's reputation? Why do the courts not just create a new legal device to achieve the desired result? Well, traditionally, courts, particularly in the United Kingdom, are reluctant to break entirely fresh ground. They are not like Haroun al Rashid sitting under a palm tree, dispensing justice. They tend towards conservatism. They prefer to move slowly, gradually, so as not to take the world by surprise. Some innovations, they think, are better left to Parliament. Of course, the precise calculation of what is for Parliament and what for them varies with time, the particular judges, and whether or not Parliament chooses to do something. The fact that courts in the United States feel less inhibited is one reason why consumerism through litigation is so much more developed there.

In the Birmingham case, the House of Lords decided that the doctor was not negligent. All this means is that the court resisted the invitation to extend the legal meaning of negligence, whatever its meaning in common speech, so as to allow the little boy to recover compensation from the doctor. The court was right to do so, not because of any question whether the doctor was at fault or not. This can be irrelevant, as we have seen, if the goal of compensating the boy is deemed socially desirable. The real reason is that if doctors were held liable, it would be their insurance which would meet the cost. But the insurance premiums paid by doctors in the United Kingdom are insufficient to meet such claims on any scale. Nor could doctors easily pay increased premiums since, within the NHS, they could not pass on the cost of such increases to patients by way of increased fees. Thus, neither party to the litigation in Birmingham ought to bear the costs of the care the little boy needed, despite the fact that we may agree he should receive it. The result was that he got nothing.

But what of the case in which the doctor was negligent, was incompetent? As I have said, this does not happen very often. But imagine it did, and money compensation beyond what the existing state system provides was needed. Does negligence litigation have a place in such a case? At present, of course, it does in the few cases in which it arises. Some argue that it should continue to do so. It keeps doctors on their toes, it is said, and probably their insurance could cover the cost. It may well be that the threat of negligence litigation is one factor which keeps doctors up to the mark. But it is manifestly unfair. It means that, at present, the person injured through negligence is compensated. The child who cannot show negligence gets nothing, though he may have suffered the same injury and has the same needs. The negligence system is concerned with how the injury is caused, rather than the fact that it has been caused. I am thus led to the view that it is necessary to separate the needs of an injured party for compensation from the need to ensure that the doctor observes certain standards of ethical behaviour and of competence.

This leads me to the third option for meeting the financial needs of the little boy and any other injured party. A fund could be created, managed by an appropriate government agency and financed from public revenue. Money would be provided as a matter of course, on proof of need. In my view this is clearly the only proper solution. There is a precedent for it in the case of the children damaged by whooping-cough vaccine, although in this case the numbers involved were admittedly small. But, only recently, in 1978, the Royal Commission on Compensation for Personal Injury rejected this view. The reason given was, inevitably, cost. But the cost arguments are not so convincing. The compensation awarded could be less than at present awarded by courts; for example, damages for pain and suffering could be eliminated. The costs now reflected in lawyers' fees and insurance costs and premiums would be saved. And novel ways of financing such a fund could be found, if the will were there. Once again, we are dealing with the need for government to make a political choice. Funds have been found for other social programmes of arguably less merit. I submit that the matter deserves reconsideration. Lord Justice Lawton echoed this view when he concluded his judgement in *Whitehouse* v. *Jordan* in the Court of Appeal by saying that 'the victims of medical mishaps of the present kind should be cared for by the community, not by the hazards of litigation'. One of England's most distinguished judges, Lord Scarman, has also lent his support to this proposition in forceful public utterances. Not surprisingly, the idea does not, however, find favour with the present Government. As the then Minister of State for Consumer Affairs put it, in the House of Commons on 4 November 1980, 'In no way would I wish to see any reform which undermined the law of tort in this country. That law is part of the fabric of society, depending as it does on the philosophy of duty and personal responsibility.' It is as if the past 50 years of development in the law, particularly in the area of insurance and social welfare, had not happened! As you can see, there is a long way to go before the argument catches up with the evidence.

My conclusion is that negligence litigation, so much a feature of American consumerism, has no place in the United Kingdom as a means of providing compensation. Let me repeat my reasons. Such litigation discriminates against certain classes of the needy, whose need may be real, but who either cannot prove someone was at fault, or were, in fact, the victims of a complete accident which was no one's fault. They must look elsewhere for the satisfaction of their needs. Secondly, it is no way to provide compensation on any scale, since the structure of medical insurance is not designed for such a task. This leads to a third point. Because money and reputation are involved, it is awfully hard to succeed in a negligence claim against a doctor. Whereas, according to the 1978 Royal Commission Report, 80–90 per cent of non-medical injury claims succeed, only 30–40 per cent of medical injury claims are successful. If contested, they are contested with energy and determination.

But does negligence litigation have a place in enforcing standards and ensuring competence? In my view it does not. The incompetent doctor does not pay any damages awarded against him if someone is harmed. His insurance company does. He is not disciplined by his professional body, so that others might not be harmed, since the General Medical Council chooses not to take jurisdiction in matters of competence. Some doctors would argue that the very fact of being sued is a sanction in itself. They talk, quite rightly, of their reputations being at stake, particularly as trials are usually widely reported. This is a considerable sanction. But, ironically, it is usually applied to those doctors who least of all those sued deserve it; that is, the doctors who are least worthy of being blamed for their conduct, if at all. This is because, in the more obvious cases of negligence, where public disapprobation would be appropriate, the case is settled out of court, and no one is the wiser. The consumer has no way of knowing about this doctor. His reputation remains intact. And, as a consequence, the consumer has no chance to exercise his option as a consumer, and avoid this doctor in the future.

Furthermore, resort to negligence actions on any scale may well drive doctors into defensive medicine. Finally, it is quite inappropriate to leave the establishment of general standards of conduct and the means of securing that they are observed to the whims of private litigation and to the lottery such litigation often proves to be. This does not mean, of course, that the consumer should not be protected from the incompetent doctor, nor that all doctors, competent or otherwise, should not be subject to review and assessment. But litigation is not the proper way.

Consumerism must take another tack. The object must be to ensure that doctors always remain accountable to the rest of society. Accountability is the key concern for the consumer. There are two issues to be resolved. Standards have to be established and made public both for technical competence and in terms of ethics. Then a proper supervisory system is needed which will ensure that these standards are observed, and appropriate sanctions exist and, if necessary, are used. The impetus will have to come from the consumer, since the medical profession seems reluctant to break out of its mould of paternalism and distrust.

As regards the establishment of ethical standards, I have already discussed this at length. As for standards of technical competence, they would be for the profession to set out, at least in the first instance. The accountants' profession is showing the way in this regard, and I believe it to be the direction all professions should follow. Such standards must be made public. Once they were published, members of the public, consumers or their advisers, would have something against which to judge the conduct of a particular case. Before the howl from the profession drowns further argument, let me remind you that the alternative, like it or not, is litigation. For the reasons I have given, I do not like it. It brings with it harrowing contests, defensiveness, a sense in the profession of being beleaguered, and a sense in the consumer of frustration. For this reason I make my proposal for a Code of Professional Standards of Competence for your consideration.

Complaints will not go away, nor will requests by patients for more information, which often are the precursors of complaints, if not sympathetically dealt with. Indeed, the overwhelming weight of evidence is that poor communication, and unwillingness to answer questions and pass on information are the breeding grounds of complaints. Teresa Smallbone, of the Consumers' Association, explained on BBC Radio in April 1981 that 'most complaints do not involve questions of skill or competence, but how the individual's case was handled'. 'Very often', she said, 'the individual is not running a vendetta against doctors or hospitals, but just wants an answer or some information.' She pointed to the evidence compiled by the Consumers' Association of 'the general tactlessness of professionals in dealing with ordinary people'. As these feelings of frustration simmer, so the risk of embitterment and a growing number of complaints grows. In their book *The British Way of Birth*, Catherine Boyd and Lea Sellers write, as Annabel Ferriman put it in her review in *The Times* of 17 March 1982, that 'a thirst for information, unsatisfied by busy or offhand staff, was frequently reported'. 'Hospital doctors were criticized for their high-handed attitude more often than general practitioners. Only 43 per cent of women said their hospital doctors were helpful and sympathetic whereas 69 per cent said their GPs were.'

Half-baked complaints procedures, such as the 1981 hospital procedure, are not enough. Both their form and the attitude they reflect of belligerent self-regulation are a recipe for further complaints, litigation and poor relations between doctor and patient. It is, quite frankly, a tragedy that those who claim to speak for the profession do not grasp this. With established Codes of Practice in ethics and in standards of competence, you have the blueprint for an understanding between the professional and the consumer, the doctor and the patient.

There would then be the question of supervising adherence to these standards and providing for the occasions on which they were breached. As regards competence, what is required is a system of interlocking mechanisms all aimed at producing compliance in the first place and, if necessary, disciplinary action. Periodic compulsory post-qualification training would be one way of ensuring that the doctor was able to maintain a proper level of competence. Peer review and audit, properly created and operated, would also have a place. A sensitive complaints procedure would be necessary, which in its form and substance demonstrated to the consumer that his interests were taken seriously. Non-professionals would have to be involved at an early stage of enquiry or review as, for example, is the case now in the legal profession. Careful training for doctors in communication skills, which would obviate many, even the majority, of complaints is, of course, essential, and far better than any complaints procedure. The Ombudsman would continue to have a role as an independent agency. With standards of competence to refer to, his brief could be extended to consider all complaints not settled at a lower, less formal level. I would also advocate the creation of an independent Professional Inspectorate which would consist of doctors whose job it was to review, on a systematic basis, the performance of doctors. Such inspectorates already exist, of course, for the police and school teachers.

All these institutions for review would have their own means of operation and would proceed by advice to, or admonition of, the consumer or the doctor. If either remained discontented, there would be recourse to a Professional Standards Review Tribunal which would bring into play a range of sanctions, from admonition to suspension, or even removal from practice. The Tribunal would be made up of a majority of non-professionals. Since the reputation and possible career of the doctor would be at stake, it would be a formal hearing, with legal representation if desired, and the right of appeal. It would not, as you can see, involve recourse to the ordinary courts nor would the enquiry into bad practice or incompetence be muddied by the fact that someone was also seeking compensation from the doctor. For, as you will recall, I have suggested that the need for compensation in the case of medical injury or accident should be dealt with separately and not be made contingent on a demonstration that the doctor behaved incompetently.

The system of review in the case of ethical propriety would be somewhat more simple. A Code of Practice, good communication and a sensitive complaints procedure would normally be enough. A Tribunal or Committee not unlike the present General Medical Council, largely consisting of non-professionals, would hear and, if necessary, impose appropriate sanctions in cases not otherwise resolved.

Solving these problems is a task with which consumerism has only just begun to grapple. It is very much a task for the future.

7 The last taboo

In this final chapter I want to pursue at greater length three issues I have already touched on: they are the role of technology in medicine and the not unrelated topics of the care of the dying and the determination of death. Let me take technology first. It warrants more consideration here because nothing epitomizes more obviously the challenge which medicine in the future faces. Resort to medical technology of ever greater complexity may have some rewards for us. But it also typifies what I have suggested is the wrong approach to the provision of medical care and the promotion of health. The question before us is how to identify and then maintain the proper balance between the good and the undesirable.

Perhaps I ought to explain that when I use the word 'technology' I have in mind the development and use of tools and machines, and the mechanical skills that go with them. Although I do not discount medicines, since they are tools, my attention will be focused primarily on mechanical tools. Some examples are the X-ray machine, the hypodermic syringe, the blood-pressure gauge and the scalpel. These have all been with us for some time. They are now deemed so necessary a part of our daily lives that to question their use would be regarded as absurd, a view I do not challenge here. Then there is the respirator, the kidney dialysis machine, the CAT scanner, which can sketch at a cost of £450,000 *per* machine a picture of the brain or other soft tissue, and the pathology laboratory's array of diagnostic equipment, complete with the latest computer. These are examples of the more recent technical paraphernalia which now are part of the armamentarium of modern medicine. It is these I shall concentrate upon. I do not think it could be said that these modern advances are different in kind from their more well-established predecessors, such as the ones I have listed. Furthermore, it may be that these predecessors in their time posed ethical questions of the kind I wish to raise. My suspicion, however, is that the ethical questions now raised by technological developments are more profoundly challenging than has ever been the case in the past, and so warrant treating modern technological innovations in medicine as qualitatively different from what has gone before.

One point must be clear. There is little sense in bemoaning, regretting or criticizing what has come to pass. There are those who regret the development of, for example, the motor car or nuclear fission. Equally, we may wish to weigh up the pros and cons and say, on balance, that we would be better off without being able to fertilize human ova in a Petri dish (the so-called test-tube baby), know the sex of a foetus long before it is due to be born, or keep the irretrievably unconscious patient in a state of suspended animation for weeks and months on end. But this is a pointless exercise. These innovations are all with us and no amount of wishful thinking will make them go away. The only fruitful exercise is to ask how what we have should be used. In this way we may regulate the future, on the lesson of the past, so as to avoid the dilemmas we now face. Even this sort of measured response and evaluation is not easy. For, as I have suggested, developments in science and technology tend to acquire a momentum of their own, such that they pass beyond ready control. Once the genie is out of the bottle, it is not a question of putting it back. That is already impossible. It is a question of making sure it does your bidding, rather than your doing its.

I have already referred to the irritating and singularly ill conceived argument of some scientists; that they are neutral researchers, seekers after knowledge. Their motives are solely concerned with truth, they argue. They cannot be held responsible for the mess mortals make of their innovations. It is always the politicians and others who are responsible for the ills which later transpire. I say this is an ill conceived argument, despite the tenacity with which it is held by the scientific establishment, for several reasons. First, a scientist is not neutral; he lives in our world and his responsibilities are to our world. He cannot detach his normative self, the part of him which makes judgements and evaluates things, from that part which conducts experiments. By pursuing research he is already making several value statements, for example that he ought to pursue research, that he ought to be allowed to pursue research, that the pursuit of research is a good thing and that the pursuit of this particular research is a good thing. Second, the assumption that knowledge and truth are some sort of ultimate deities, the worship of which guarantees a lasting state of grace in the worshipper, cannot go without challenge. There are countless examples where knowledge and truth are not pursued because the pursuit would challenge values we hold more dear than them. In other words, knowledge and truth as conceived of by the scientist are not necessarily, or always, the ultimate values in our society. Take for example someone who wished to carry out an experiment which was potentially life-threatening. Would we countenance his experimenting on, for example, prisoners, or consenting participants, or even, if we had them, killers condemned to die? The answer is that we, or most of us, would not. Certain values we will not compromise with, even if the cry is heard that this is standing in the way of the pursuit of knowledge. Indeed, to choose an albeit extreme example, Karl Brandt, who was responsible for much of the human experimentation which took place in the concentration camps, was hanged after the Second World War because he chose not to observe these first principles in his pursuit of knowledge. It was as a consequence of this trial that the Nuremberg Code of 1947 was drafted to regulate the conduct of research on human subjects. The 1964 Declaration of Helsinki, revised in 1975, is the latest statement of principle.

Despite the strength of such arguments against the simplistic notion of the value-free scientist who should be left to pursue knowledge and technical innovation, the pursuit goes on. Of course, it is not unbridled and limitations are set as to what ought to be done. To that extent scientists speak out of the other corner of their mouths, and point to the ethical codes under which they work, notwithstanding that theirs is a value-free exercise. But, of course, if an outsider, a non-scientist, concerns himself with such ethical codes, he is, as we have seen, quickly reminded that he is trespassing on the scientists' preserve. This involves an argument which changes sides half-way along, for if matters of ethics are involved it is open for all to comment.

Thus, the momentum of scientific and technological development which I spoke of persists and is extremely difficult to check without attracting the universal odium of the scientific establishment. And this is as true in medicine as in other areas. For example, the continued pursuit of more and more complicated diagnostic tools goes on as if in a vacuum, insulated from questions such as whether the growing expense justifies the exercise, or whether being able to identify certain physical phenomena is particularly worthwhile if once they are identified little can be done to tag them with the appropriate label.

There has appeared in medicine the well-known phenomenon which I have called the technological imperative — if you can do it, you ought to do it. Thus, the mere existence of equipment dictates that it be used. As we have seen, this is attractive to the doctor trained to think of himself as the problem-solver and applied scientist. Furthermore, it serves to justify the purchase of the equipment. If you have recently fitted out a modern intensive care unit, you will want to use it, both to prove how essential it was and because not to use it may now be thought to be neglect of the patient. You see the cycle developing momentum. The innovator develops the equipment, the producer needs to sell it, so appeals to the latent engineer or scientist in the doctor. The doctor recommends it be acquired and once it is acquired feels compelled to use it. That it may not have been necessary, that it serves to perpetuate an unfortunate model of medicine and the pursuit of health, that it attracts resources away from areas where greater benefit to health may be achieved, that patients do not seem to gain a great deal from it, that operational errors are made — all these and more are lost in the technological imperative.

How should we respond to this? First, we must notice that there are two important factors to be weighed in considering technological innovation in medicine. They are the implications, first, in terms of resources expended, and, second, in terms of ethical problems posed. I do not wish to dwell here on resources, but given the finite amount of money and manpower available for health care it is clear that some analysis in terms of costs and benefits is called for. These analyses, however, are notoriously hard to carry out. It is not easy to demonstrate that spending £x to treat 1,000 patients a year whereby 150 have their life expectancy considerably increased is less justified than spending it on putting fluoride in drinking water so that the incidence of dental caries is drastically reduced, or less justified than spending the same amount of money in wiping out the waiting-list for hernia operations so that working men may return to work. The problem becomes even more difficult when one recalls that any analysis must be seen in the light of the changing fads and fashions of medicine, whereby a particular innovation is first greeted enthusiastically, then later challenged or abandoned, and then sometimes taken up again, such as the transplantation of such organs as the liver or lungs or even the heart, or the massive care devoted to all babies born with spina bifida. Further, such analysis must take account of the politics of medicine, whereby the consultant in the teaching hospital has his hands on more levers of power than do others.

Certainly, such cost-benefit analyses must be carried out despite their difficulty. A considerable number of studies have already been undertaken, particularly in the United States, though the field is relatively new as a rigorous exercise rather than a hit-and-miss affair. Unfortunately, many of the studies are flawed. Most, for example, have been carried out by economists who, perhaps, lack the necessary training and insight to take account of the competing moral and spiritual values involved. Their work, therefore, is at best a partial guide and leaves unanswered the various ethical problems which call for resolution. Gavin Mooney, Director of the Health Economics Research Unit at Aberdeen University, stoutly defends cost-benefit analyses in the *Journal of Medical Ethics* of December 1980. They are, he concedes, separate from any consideration of medical ethics, but they can reveal inefficiencies and irrationalities of policies directed towards certain goals. One difficulty with such an argument is that efficiency, consistency, or rationality are in themselves ethical principles which may not always be acceptable if, in the pursuit of them, other values deemed more worthwhile are ignored. Other cost-benefit analyses have been undertaken by those with axes to grind, so that the results tend to be self-serving. For how you value a life or a limb or a limp may well be a product of the particular proposal you are making, since it is hard to argue that they have any constant and objective value. As Professor Guido Calabresi, of Yale Law School, has pointed out, we make rather curious social decisions concerning risks. For example, we may choose not to install a traffic light at an intersection despite the relatively low cost and the annual two or three deaths at the intersection caused by colliding cars. We may, on the other hand, choose to spend large sums, relatively speaking, to search for and rescue some mountain climber who has been fool enough to go climbing in a blizzard.

Muir Gray makes the point well by referring to the 1978 study conducted by the Office of Health Economics. Under the heading of 'Values of life inferred from several public policy decisions', he cites the following table, drawn from the study:

Decision	Implied value of life	Comment and source
Not to introduce child-proof drug containers	£1,000 maximum	In 1971 the Government decided not to proceed with the child-proofing of drug containers.
Legislation on tractor cabs	£100,000 minimum	In 1969 the fitting of cabs to farm tractors, to reduce mortality risk to drivers was made compulsory. The cost per annum was estimated at £4 million (£40 for each of 100,000 tractors). About 40 lives would be saved annually.
Changes in building regulations as a result of partial collapse of Ronan Point high-rise flats	£20,000,000 minimum or perhaps actual	After a high-rise block of flats partially collapsed, killing some residents, the report of the inquiry recommended changes in the building standards of such blocks. It has been estimated from the change in risk and the cost involved that the implied value of life was £20 million.
Not to provide treatment for chronic renal failure for a person aged 50	£30,000 (Office of Health Economics estimate 1976-7 prices)	Particularly in regions where facilities are in short supply, a person over the age of 45 or 50 may stand little chance of being accepted for treatment by dialysis or transplantation.

Clearly, there is much to be done here before we can make intelligent choices based on an understanding of the implications, in terms of resources, of the development and introduction of medical technology.

Now let me turn to the ethical implications. There cannot be any doubt that very many of the ethical problems which dog modern medicine can be traced to technological developments. Take the example of kidney dialysis. About 5,000 people each year in the United Kingdom fall victim to kidney failure. Access to a dialysis machine means life to those whose kidneys fail, but calls for the awful and awesome decision as to who is to receive the benefit of a machine, when demand outstrips supply. In a parliamentary reply on 2 June 1980, the Secretary of State told Parliament that about 1,100 people were able to begin dialysis in 1978, an increase from 600 in 1971. The figure remains at about this level. But despite an increase in the number of successful kidney transplant operations performed, this still means that hundreds will still die each year from kidney failure. The question arises of how many machines ought to be made available when they cost about £6,000 to buy and between £8,000 and £12,000 each year to operate. Furthermore, the difficult question arises as to what the proper relationship between dialysis and transplants should be. Should a patient whose transplant fails, automatically have access again to a dialysis machine? These are just a few of the ethical problems related to dialysis, there are many others.

The recital of ethical problems is equally long and complex when other technological innovations are considered. There is, for example, the mass screening of women for breast cancer. The screening may itself be harmful. Furthermore, the discovery of the tumour may not significantly affect the mortality of the woman, although it may on occasions increase the sum of her unhappiness by causing her to know that much earlier. There is the elaborate technology of life support which has served to reinforce our unwillingness to admit death. There is transplant surgery. A question concerning the transplanting of vital organs which still awaits an answer is whether it is justified in terms of the results produced, leaving aside any consideration of cost.

Equally difficult is the question of the circumstances under which organs may be removed, whether from the dead or the living. For example, should the law in the United Kingdom be changed to allow, in the case of organs removed from the dead, the routine salvaging of viable organs without the need for consent of anyone, unless the dead person had registered an objection during his lifetime? This is the solution I advocate, as long as we continue to endorse such surgery. It would favour the interests of those who may otherwise die. But it would do so only at the cost of ignoring the strongly held views of some who believe a corpse should be inviolate, and express concern that a person may not, for whatever reason, have registered an objection, yet may be opposed to his body being used for transplant purposes. The feelings of relatives of a deceased person could also be deeply hurt if organs from his body were removed without their knowledge or leave. This difference is reflected by the expressions 'opting in', which is the present English law, and 'opting out', which allows organs to be taken without consent and is the law in a number of European countries, for example, France, Austria and Denmark. Numerous efforts have been made to change the law, the Human Tissue Act, since it was passed in 1961, but all have so far failed. The legislative debates reflect the tension between the ethical principle of respecting the dignity of the dead and relatives, and that of doing good for the living and seeking to achieve justice for them. So far, the former principle has prevailed.

The problems are no more simple in the case of donations of organs by the living. Obviously the first point is that a living person may not donate an organ vital to his continued existence, such as his heart. This is not an idle point since examples exist of parents or relatives or even strangers offering vital organs for transplant. An early example reported in *The Times* of 20 August 1968 was of volunteers prepared to offer their hearts for transplant into ex-President Eisenhower who was at that point near to death. Some would argue that donations of major organs (clearly blood in appropriate measure presents no problems) by the living should never be countenanced, despite the apparent consent of the donor, because such consent can never really be valid. The donor is usually a close relative of the patient. Under such circumstances, the pressure, conscious or unconscious, applied by family, friends or even the patient make any notion of voluntariness unrealistic. The donor may indeed later feel bitter or resentful at having been put in a situation in which he felt he had no choice.

The issue of consent is particularly difficult in the case of children. Should the parents of a ten-year-old child be allowed to consent on his behalf to his donating a kidney to his young brother? I find myself unable to support the argument that such a consent is valid. Ordinarily, the law stipulates that parents may only consent to that which is in the particular child's best interests. Courts in the United States, particularly in the unreported cases in Massachusetts which preceded the first kidney transplants in 1954, have persuaded themselves that the removal of a healthy kidney from a healthy child may indeed be in the child's best interests. The reason offered is that the child will benefit psychologically from knowing that he has saved his brother, whereas he would otherwise be grief-stricken. The high point of this reasoning can be found in the Kentucky case of *Strunk* v. *Strunk*, (445 SW 2d 145, 1969) in which the court allowed the removal of a kidney from a 27-year-old with an alleged mental age of six for transplant into his 26-year-old brother on the ground that the donor 'was greatly dependant on [his brother] emotionally and psychologically and that his well-being would be jeopardized more severely by the loss of his brother than the removal of his kidney'. I find this reasoning most unpersuasive. I take the view that until a child reaches an age at which he may make an informed and mature decision for himself, surgery of this kind should not be performed.

Indeed, it is salutary to contrast this approach with that adopted in the case of *McFall* v. *Shimp*, decided in Pennsylvania in 1978 and well described in Russell Scott's book, *The Body as Property*. Robert McFall was dying of aplastic anaemia. His cousin, David Shimp, agreed to undergo a test which was to show that his bone marrow was a perfect match for McFall. Pinning all his hopes on a bone marrow transplant, McFall then discovered that Shimp had decided not to become involved any further. In desperation, McFall asked a court to order his cousin to give up his bone marrow. The court refused, reasoning that to compel Shimp 'would defeat the sanctity of the individual and would impose a rule that would know no limits'. 'One human being', the judge went on, 'cannot legally be compelled to aid another.' Acts of what the moral philosophers call supererogation, where there is no duty to act, are for the individual alone to make. Of course, this is partly question-begging, since it is always possible to convert what was regarded as an act of supererogation – for example, rescuing a drowning man – into a duty, as has happened in a number of European legal systems. Quite whether someone should be forced to undergo surgery for his neighbour is hard to decide, but I suspect that we have not heard the last of the argument. Three weeks after he lost his case in court, McFall died.

Finally, in this list of examples of ethical difficulties arising out of technological innovation, there is the tightrope walk of chemo-therapy. Used to treat tumours, the line between killing the patient and killing a part of him is so narrow that Senator Hubert Humphrey was moved to describe his treatment for cancer of the bladder, from which he eventually died, as 'chemical death'.

I could go on. All these are agonizingly difficult ethical dilemmas, but it is another unfortunate and disquieting consequence of their arising out of the practice of advanced technology medicine that, because they are a consequence of the use of technical measures, they are treated as questions for the technical expert, the doctor, to decide. They are another species of the ethical question treated as a medical matter and therefore properly for the doctor alone to decide which I examined earlier. Once again it it obvious that this view cannot be sustained. A doctor has no more competence than you or I to decide, for example, which of competing candidates should have access to a kidney machine in the context of a scarcity of resources. The answer will be offered that the kidney machine goes to the patient medically most suited, but this is patently question-begging, particularly when such factors as psychological stability and ability to comprehend and follow the necessary regime of food and behaviour are considered. Clearly, doctors must be the arbiters of those questions which are technical. Thereafter, the issue is an ethical one, even including the question of how far such technical information is to be deemed relevant to the conclusion to be reached. It may be that the solution which is least objectionable is a lottery, though many would object. A lottery was for instance used to allocate polio vaccine in England when it was first introduced and supplies were scarce. Of course, any lottery would exclude those who, because of, for example, other illness, were in the strictest sense medically unsuitable. It is no answer to say that the real solution is the provision of enough machines for all, since this itself is part of a larger question concerning the allocation of resources among competing claims. It is in the resolution of such problems that a Code of Practice on medical ethics is so urgently required.

Victor Parsons and P. Lock show in the study I mentioned earlier, published in the *Journal of Medical Ethics* of December 1980, that the decisions which have to be made at present are agonizingly difficult for doctors. It seems quite unfair to place doctors in such a position. Their study consisted of a questionnaire sent to twenty-five renal dialysis units in the United Kingdom. Each unit was given the particulars of forty patients and told that ten would have to be rejected. Parsons and Lock write that many of the doctors 'wrote long qualifying letters expressing their anxiety'. 'Only one physician', they report, 'felt unable to reject any of the patients suggested on medical grounds.' In the event, the results of the study were that 'only 13 patients out of forty, i.e., one third, stood the chance of being accepted in all the units questioned; on the other hand no single patient in the series was rejected by all unit physicians. When we came to analyse the ten patients most frequently rejected, we found that at least six of them had been successfully treated by our own unit' (the cases were each based on real clinical practice).

H.J.J.Lennen, in the *Journal of Medical Ethics* of March 1982, argues against a lottery and tries to suggest another way of solving the dilemma illustrated by Parsons and Lock. His proposal is most constructive. It suggests that criteria which are as free from subjective evaluation as possible be relied on, in a descending order of importance. He discards criteria such as age, or social behaviour or social worth as too untrustworthy. He would leave the decision as to whether the patient fits within these pre-established criteria to the doctor treating him. Here you have the beginnings of a defensible solution. Lennen's ideas warrant careful consideration.

It is fair to say, however, that some deny that the problem exists, despite the volume of literature about it. A study of three regions, undertaken through the auspices of the Royal College of Physicians, and published in the *British Medical Journal* of 25 July 1981, suggests there is no problem. 'While the criteria varied', the Report asserts, 'the reasons given for non-acceptance of cases [for dialysis or transplant] seemed sound, and in no instance . . . was a patient denied dialysis because of a shortage of machines.' Certainly, the Report is justified in making the point, which is often overlooked, that some cases are, unfortunately, medically unsuitable and beyond the help of dialysis, because of the nature of the illness involved. But I venture to suggest that the study warrants careful attention. It was confined to deaths in hospital of those under 50 years of age. This, of course, eliminates from consideration those over 50, a group who encounter renal failure and who, according to the 1982 London area study I mentioned earlier, do not have access to dialysis. In Germany, France and Italy, according to this 1982 study, three times more patients between 55 and 64 are treated than in the United Kingdom, and 15 times more in the age range 65–74. Then, when the reasons given in the Royal College's Report are examined, it may be questioned whether they necessarily support the conclusion. For example, the following reasons were offered to those compiling the Report for not offering dialysis (the authors remarked, you will recall, that they 'seemed sound'): 'Unco-operative patient. Dialysis requested by physician but deemed inappropriate by nephrologist'; or, 'Question of dialysis not raised'; or, 'Very unintelligent. Dialysis not mentioned'; or, 'Spoke no English. Pulmonary tuberculosis. Psychological instability'; or, 'Spina bifida. Very little leg movement'. It will come as no surprise that the Report was not without its critics. I remain convinced, in accordance with the leading article in the *Lancet* of 14 March 1981, that decisions as to whom to treat rest on resources rather than on clinical criteria.

A further ethical implication of the resort to advanced technology in medicine is the effect it may have on the way medicine and the doctor–patient relationship are conceived of by the doctor. The machine interposes itself between the doctor and the patient. It is relied upon. Any errors or misfortunes are its doing. Successes are the doctor's. The graveyard humour of 'the operation was a success but the patient died' takes on a new significance when it is argued that the technique is perfectly sound but the patient did not respond to treatment. The applied scientist model is reinforced at the expense of the model of the caring partner. Indeed, the machine may even become the end in itself, the *raison d'être* of the doctor, so that we may be persuaded to screen everyone for a susceptibility to a particular illness or abnormality without being in any way able to do anything with the information gained. In passing, it is interesting to wonder whether we are not seeing social history repeating itself here. Modern medicine, as we have seen, finds itself faced by and large with intractable conditions for which it can offer palliative measures at best. The days of conquest and cure on any large scale are gone. We are in a sense back in the state we were in before the major eradication of infectious diseases in the nineteenth and early twentieth centuries. Technology may be our modern witchcraft. We place the machine between us and the person complaining of being ill. The expert is trusted and relied upon. Sometimes the person gets well or improves, and we praise the wonders of technology. Sometimes he does not and we reassure ourselves that we did our best. I do not push the metaphor too far, but I offer it as worth consideration.

We have already considered ways of responding to the kind of ethical dilemmas I have alluded to. Put in its simplest form, we, as ordinary people, must exercise some control. Those who develop and apply technology in medicine must be held accountable to all of us. I interject immediately that by control I do not mean prohibition or some heavy-handed bureaucratic machine. I mean that some mechanism must be created and established which is independent of any particular interest. Its role must be to lay down guidelines by reference to which the appropriate ethical decisions can be made. The crucial first task of this independent body would be to call for and disseminate information. By and large, the ethical problems we face are a consequence of technology being developed and introduced without any general awareness. What I contemplate is measured debate both before research is undertaken and before technology is introduced. This can only take place if information, on what is being done and what it may involve, is available to all. And in this context, as in many others, information is power, the first necessary step towards control.

The question then arises as to how a body such as the one I have suggested, on which an appropriately broad spectrum of opinion will be represented, will exercise control. No one wants to see Government, or medicine, by committee. What I envisage is that after the first task, that of informing, is accomplished, issues of a general nature will be laid before this body of people and there debated. Comments would be invited from interested persons. Then guidelines would be produced which would serve as operating criteria according to which the research could be undertaken or the technology put into operation. It may be objected that this is a rather elaborate and slow process. But it is not beyond the wit of man to build a system which can operate successfully. Furthermore, time taken to debate the opening of the bottle is well spent if it means that the evil genie stays inside. The inquiry in 1978 into the siting of a nuclear power station conducted by Mr Justice Parker allowed the whole future of the use of nuclear energy in the United Kingdom to be debated and provides a model. That all did not approve of the final decisions does not invalidate the success of the enterprise. And of course such a large inquiry would be the exception rather than the rule, necessary when matters of the greatest significance for the future were involved.

Let me now turn to the dilemmas of modern medicine surrounding the end of life. I will concentrate on two issues – caring for the dying and the determination of death. It must be one of the most banal of statements to say that we must all die. But it seems sometimes as if we need to be reminded of the fact. *The Times* of 14 December 1976 heralded public discussion of death and dying as breaking 'The last taboo'. But the taboo is far from broken. It could be said that our interest is that of the voyeur and it co-exists with that other part of our modern way of thinking, the denial of death, or at least the refusal to give it much thought, as being something that happens to others. The voyeur in us, for example, makes world-wide news of such common-place tragedies as that of Karen Quinlan, just another girl who, through drugs or alcohol or both, ended up on a respirator in hospital. But that part of us which denies the inevitability of death prevents us from examining the facts, analysing what ought to be done, and suggesting remedies. We are content to say 'poor thing' and wait for the next news item.

This sort of ambivalence is most obvious in the United States where there has been such an amazing outpouring of books, papers, news-paper articles and television programmes about death and dying, that it may be one of the liveliest growth industries in American letters. Yet, alongside this, the latest fad to preserve life, whether it be ginseng or jogging, sends this same middle-class voyeur off on another pursuit of Xanadu. Clinging to life reaches its high point in the lunatic fringe's conversion to cryogenics, whereby people are frozen after death to await some cure for that which killed them. Do not blame me for the logic. I am just repeating the argument. Jessica Mitford's biting commentary in *The American Way of Death* has not lost its validity. If anything has changed, it is merely that the death industry has become more respectable and intellectualized.

Perhaps the most important insight into the process of caring for the dying is that dying has become, to many, an illness. Call some-thing an illness and you convert it into something which may respond to treatment, can even, perhaps, be cured. Add to this the doctor's claim that you cannot be sure that someone is dying — 'he may recover, others have' — and you set the scene for a medical denial of death to complement the layman's. Death becomes like illness and disease, something to be defeated. The battle is not lost while there is something more which can be done. This is the point. We are in danger of seeing dying as something the doctor has to do something about, to try to prevent. We tend to expect this as an extension of our own anxieties and by medicalizing dying the doctor is trapped by his own claim to expertise. Since a very large proportion of those who die do so now in hospital, this process of the medicalization of death has inevitably gained momentum. Indeed, being in hospital the dying person confronts a medical attitude which will inevitably reflect the values of medicine which I have been describing. For, in general, it is the hospital doctor who *par excellence* considers himself the applied scientist and problem-solver. There is a danger that dying comes to be seen as just another problem to be solved. Death is in a real sense a failure, not to be allowed without a fight. And, when you add into the equation the existence of the paraphernalia of modern life support technology, you supply the doctor with the tools with which to act out this communal denial of death.

It was Professor Henry Miller who railed against the sight of elderly patients existing in the twilight zone between life and death but not allowed to cross into the shadow because of the wonders of modern medicine. In the *Proceedings* of the Royal Society of Medicine of November 1967, Professor Miller wrote that 'there must be very few doctors who have not from time to time felt uneasiness, if not revulsion, at the spectacle of some stuporous ancient in hospital being maintained in a state of suspended animation by all the sophisticated paraphernalia of modern resuscitation'.

There has more recently been some conscious effort to move away from this unsightly exercise and to change the attitude of doctors and lay people. The Hospice Movement has grown up, pioneered by Dame Cicely Saunders. Patients enter the hospice to await death. The regime is one of care which emphasizes concern for the spiritual and psychological state of the patient but sets its face against the kind of technological warfare traditional hospitals may indulge in. Crucially, the staff concentrate on easing any pain the dying person may have, whether physical or mental. Years of research with mood-elevating drugs and with drugs to ease pain and control unpleasant symptoms have produced a body of pharmacotherapeutic knowledge which leads hospice staff to argue that no one now need die in pain or misery. This may be true in theory and the 'Brompton cocktail', a mixture of strong pain-killing drugs under the influence of which the patient slid to his death, should be a thing of the past. The harsh fact, however, is that the vast majority of dying people do not find their way into hospices. Rather they die in general hospitals, often only after all efforts have been exhausted, where the careful management of pain and attention to spiritual needs hospice-style is unlikely to be encountered. Those involved in hospice care, in particular Robert Twycross at Oxford, whose skill and compassion are an example to all, argue strongly that we do not need more hospices. What we do need as a matter of urgency, and what he and others like him work energetically towards, is the dissemination of the skills and knowledge acquired in the hospices out to the general hospitals.

The principal ethical issue involved in the care of the dying concerns the duty the doctor owes his patient once the view is reached that the patient is dying. Note that I put the question in the form of the doctor's duty. This is because in my view the key concept in understanding the ethical basis of the doctor–patient relationship is duty, a duty owed by the doctor to the patient. Now I know some will say that I beg the question by assuming that the patient is dying, whereas the doctor may not be able to know this with such assurance. I readily concede that there must be a grey area in which the prognosis for the patient cannot be stated with precision. At the same time I would argue that if the doctor were making his determination in good faith, free of the pressure of others, whether relatives, nurses or colleagues, and liberated from the self-image of himself as the problem-solver to whom death is failure, the view that a particular patient is dying can indeed be arrived at in very many cases. In the hope of avoiding confusion let me offer a further clarification. There are of course patients whose illness is fatal but who are at present enjoying a remission or are still able to live their lives albeit within narrowing constraints. I exclude these from those I refer to here as dying. I have in mind instead those whose illness has reached a terminal stage and for whom remission is either no longer possible or bought at great cost in terms of suffering or hardship.

Once a patient is seen to be dying, the duty the doctor owes him is, in my view, best stated as the duty to make what remains of his life comfortable. This is the principal ethical and legal duty. It carries with it the counterpart that the doctor has a duty to desist from measures which are designed to do other than comfort the patient. Continued chemotherapy, for example, or radiotherapy in the case of a dying patient, accompanied as they are by discomfort, are not only uncalled for but a breach of the doctor's duty to his patient. The doctor does not desist from treating his patient. What changes is the nature of the treatment which is provided. His care is no longer for the living. He must now care for the dying.

Seen in this light, a question which fascinates so many, that of when it is proper to turn off a respirator, can be shown to be one of the more simple questions to answer and it may be worth dealing with it here in passing. You must place the patient on the respirator into one of four categories. The first comprises those patients who are dead. The respirator is merely filling a corpse with air. Provided the determination of death is properly made, something I shall consider shortly, the respirator can be turned off. In the second category is the person who needs the respirator to breathe and is irreversibly unconscious. Once the patient's condition is incontrovertibly established, the doctor must, from time to time, disconnect the patient from the respirator so as to test the ability of the patient to breathe for himself. If the patient can breathe for himself, the question then becomes one of keeping him comfortable. Should he then develop some infection such as pneumonia the doctor is entitled to decide that given the hopelessness of the patient's condition he is not obliged to intervene to treat the infection but that his duty is rather to let the patient die. If, however, the patient does not breathe for himself or does so in a manner which would not be consistent with remaining alive, the doctor is entitled to consider whether returning the patient to the respirator is called for. If the patient's condition is so irreversibly hopeless, the doctor is entitled to desist from returning him to the respirator. The doctor is not obliged to continue with measures which are pointless and hopeless in that the patient's condition shows no possibility of recovery or improvement. The ethical question thus becomes not one of turning off the respirator but rather of turning it back on again. A third class of patient consists of those for whom the prognosis is still in doubt or who, for the time being, for whatever reason, need the respirator to aid breathing. In these circumstances, the doctor's duty is to persist with the respirator until the patient recovers, improves, or reaches the stage in which the prognosis is hopeless. If it is hopeless, the respirator is a burden and an intrusion upon the patient, as in the previous case, and the doctor, having turned it off to ascertain the patient's condition, is entitled to desist from turning it back on. The final class consists of those patients who are fully conscious and otherwise competent but who for reasons of some illness, for example polio, cannot breathe for themselves. There can be no question here of turning off the respirator as it cannot be classified as a hopeless and burdensome imposition on a patient who but for the respirator would die a peaceful death. From this brief outline it can be seen that the ethically relevant decision is not whether to turn off the respirator. Rather, it is the decision whether to put the patient on the respirator, or to turn it back on again having turned it off, in the light of the prognosis.

The ethical duty of the doctor, therefore, in general terms, moves from the duty to maintain and preserve life to the duty to make the patient comfortable and avoid all intervention of a pointless and hopeless nature. This movement coincides with that of the patient from being categorized as ill and therefore capable of recovery or improvement, or at least not dying, to being categorized as dying. However, a powerful combination of factors all conspire to produce a situation in which the dying are not easily allowed to die. They include the training of doctors as problem-solvers, our cultural rejection or denial of death, pressure from relatives or, rarely, patients themselves, the existence of the technology to maintain a semblance of life and the enthusiasm, particularly of young doctors, to regard dying as a challenge to be overcome. 'Rage, rage against the dying of the light' was how Dylan Thomas captured our inability to come to terms with death. The unseemly intervention of doctors, flown in from all over the world, in the dying agony of such figures as General Franco, President Tito and the Shah of Iran, and the morbid attention given to this by the press, radio and television, serve to reinforce this attitude.

It is no wonder that there have appeared movements concerned with 'Death with Dignity' or 'The Right to Die'. This latter label is, of course, rather silly. Those supporting it do not really call for a right to die. We all die, right or no. What they really mean is the right to be allowed to die without further medical intervention. They would remind us of the ethical principle of respect for dignity. They call for the ultimate right to self-determination and control, the right to have your own death. It is no wonder either that there is renewed interest in voluntary euthanasia and in suicide, even to the point of a proposal we noted earlier by the organization in the United Kingdom called Exit to publish a pamphlet for members containing instructions on effective self-destruction. The fear of languishing in the twilight state between life and death, as a medical preparation, a tribute to medical technology, is an important factor in bringing this about. Remove the fear, reassert the true nature of the doctor's duty and the need would disappear.

Of course, it is only right to notice that doctors often find themselves in an unenviable situation. Their view of their duty to the patient may be challenged by relatives who demand all efforts to be continued, hopeless though they may be. The doctor is damned if he continues and thereby breaches his duty. But he is damned if he does not, since the relatives may apply pressure, complain or even threaten him with a lawsuit for neglecting his patient. The problem is that it is hard to find any authoritative statement of society's decision as to the doctor's duty, whether in the form of law or otherwise. This lack of any clear guide allows the dilemmas I have identified to persist. I have no doubt that what I have said represents both the ethical and legal duty of the doctor. But clearly there is a need to state this view in some authoritative form. I would not have thought that this was a matter for the heavy hand of legislation, or even for a ruling in a case brought before the courts, although both solutions have been tried in the United States. Instead, it should form part of the Code of Practice I have urged upon you. Doctors' jealous defence of what they mistakenly regard as their sphere of exclusive competence and the traditionally British attitude of muddling through have combined so far to prevent this from happening. But, if the price to be paid is unhappiness and misery and if the doctor has so much to gain from the help such a Code would offer, it would be better if something were done and done soon.

I turn now to the definition and determination of death. It is a commonplace now that the modern medical technology of intensive care and life support has rendered the old ways of recognizing death unreliable. It used to be said that death was the absence of vital functions. The vital functions which were thought to be particularly relevant were breathing, heartbeat and the capacity for consciousness. Now we all know that breathing and heartbeat can be maintained by machinery, so that this way of determining death may not be helpful in the case of patients who find themselves in intensive care units. It may not be the patient who is breathing. The patient may have suffered such irreversible damage as to be unable ever to breathe again. It may be the machine which is breathing for the patient. The machine may, in a word, mimic life. The question is how to analyse this intellectually, and how to discover it in fact.

Clearly, it is important to know when and whether someone is dead. Not only does he cease to be a person but our attitude to him changes completely. He is a corpse not a person. A doctor owes a corpse no duties, save perhaps decent respect. A corpse has no claims on anyone, nor any obligations. A living person is owed duties and can have obligations. The law of homicide calls for a dead body. The law of succession comes into operation only on death. We only bury people when they are dead. And, of limited importance, but crucial in focusing attention on the issue of death, we may not remove the vital organs of someone for the purposes of transplantation until that person is dead. Kidneys and other organs must be removed fairly soon after death (within about an hour) if they are to be of use when transplanted. Not surprisingly, there was some sense of unease, especially in the early days, particularly of heart transplants, that maybe some medical sleight-of-hand was being practised. The need to determine the moment of death, hitherto not regarded as particularly crucial since time was no longer of the essence, became of the greatest significance.

There are in fact two problems involved in any analysis of the meaning of death. The first concerns the definition of death; the second, the determination that the state as defined is present. Let us consider the definition first. It cannot be stated too emphatically that the definition of death, the question what does death mean, is not for medical scientists or doctors alone to answer. What death means is the product of views on life. The word death only has significance if it is used as a counterpoise to life. So, we are really interested in the meaning of life. We are asking, when does life leave someone? Put another way, when does someone cease to be a person? A person is someone whom the law protects, to whom duties are owed both legal and ethical, and who may make claims on others. What we are concerned with is the identification of that which is crucial to being a person. This is clearly a philosophical and spiritual issue. Scientific information is relevant in helping us to analyse the concept of personality. But it cannot, of itself, tell us what personality consists of. This calls for a judgement. The definition of death calls, therefore, for a normative judgement. It calls for the selection of a point beyond which we are prepared to say someone is no longer a person.

To speak of the selection of a point is to understand that a number of options might exist in a process that begins with birth. We could say that someone is no longer a person, is dead, only when he has completely and totally decomposed. We could say someone is dead when he is unconscious, in a coma from which he will never recover, even though he is still breathing. If consciousness were the key, we could say that someone who was so severely mentally retarded as to display no evidence of conscious awareness, or someone in an advanced state of senility, is dead. In mediaeval times, it may be recalled, entering the church was described as civil death. The person no longer existed according to the civil law.

Of the various choices available, the point at which death is deemed to occur has always been that point at which the vital functions of breathing, heartbeat and the capacity for consciousness have ceased for ever. This may have been because the heart was once regarded as the seat of the emotions and it was these which were identified as being the crucial feature of being a person. The heart is no longer thought of as being the seat of the emotions, except perhaps by the manufacturers of Valentine cards. The brain has supplanted it as that part of us in which are thought to reside the mind, the emotions, the spiritual sense of self. This might lead us to abandon heartbeat and breathing as the relevant criteria of personality, and thus of life and death, in favour of consciousness. But the difficulty with this is that consciousness can be lost for ever, but a person in such a condition may continue to breathe. This is because breathing and heartbeat do not depend for their continued functioning on that part of the brain responsible for conscious thought, the higher brain. Rather, it is the brain-stem, that part at the base and back of the brain, which is responsible for their continued functioning. So, if we were to regard permanent loss of consciousness as death, it would mean that someone would be dead who was breathing of his own accord. Clearly, this is unacceptable and the importance of the old notion of absence of vital functions, breathing, heartbeat, and capacity for consciousness, reasserts itself. This has led some to argue for a definition of death which calls for the destruction of the higher brain *and* the brain-stem, so-called total brain death, as this would seem to take account of all the vital functions.

The notion of being a person shifted, therefore, from the heart to the total brain. But there is something wrong with this analysis. It does not carry the thinking through to the logical end. This is because, you see, the brain-stem is not only responsible for maintaining breathing and heartbeat. It is also responsible for the continued capacity to function of the higher brain in which consciousness resides. The brain-stem is akin to the body's switchboard. All signals go through it. If it is destroyed, nothing can function. There can be no breathing, no heartbeat, no thought. Thus, what is crucial to personality is the brain-stem, not the total brain, since it is the brain-stem which maintains all vital functions. Death on this basis, therefore, is the total and irreversible loss of all brain-stem function. The progression, intellectually, has been from heart to brain to brain-stem. Furthermore, this definition does no violence to the traditional notion of death, the absence of vital functions. All it does is to allow the absence of these functions to be identified when otherwise they may be thought still to exist because a patient is being maintained on a respirator which is breathing for him, at least temporarily, and making his heart beat.

Some are uneasy about this notion of death. They are reluctant to make the step from total brain death to brain-stem death. They persist in the view that the upper brain must be shown to be completely devoid of all electrical activity before someone can be regarded as dead. This view, in the opinion of many, is unwarranted. It fails to take account of the fact that the upper brain's ability to function is dependent on the brain-stem. And it argues for a new meaning of death.

Let me explain this second criticism. What concerns those who argue for total brain death is that even when the destruction of the brain-stem can be established, it is still possible on occasions to monitor, with the use of an electroencephalograph, electrical activity in the higher brain. Only when this activity has ceased for ever, they argue, should a person be regarded as dead. The objection to this line of argument is that what is being monitored is spontaneous electrical activity which may well persist after the death of a person. After all, the hair and finger nails of a corpse will continue to grow after death. We do not wait until they have stopped growing before declaring death. Nor do we need to wait for every trace of electrical discharge in the higher brain to have disappeared. To do so would confuse the death of a person with the subsequent death of parts of his body, in this case his higher brain, which we have already noticed cannot have the capacity to be conscious once the brain-stem is destroyed. It would mean that a new notion of death, quite distinct from the notion of absence of vital functions, was being advocated.

Clearly, if brain-stem death represented in fact a *new* notion of death, it would not be for doctors or medical scientists to decide upon and adopt it. Given that death represents a fundamental judgement about the nature of life and personality, it would be for all of us to debate and discuss before any new definition were accepted. But, for the reasons I have given, I do not regard brain-stem death as a new definition of death. Rather, I see it as a way of clarifying what we have always regarded as death, made necessary by the fact that machines can now mimic life. It is the relatively small number of adherents of total brain death who are in fact advocating a new definition of death, even though they purport to be defending the traditional definition. Their view has been rejected, at least in the United Kingdom. In 1976 the Royal Colleges of Medicine endorsed the concept of brain-stem death, reaffirming that it was no more than another way of expressing the traditional notion of death as being the absence of vital functions.

In the United States, however, there is still an unwillingness to make the intellectual step from total brain death to brain-stem death. Indeed, in its lengthy and detailed study, *Defining Death*, published in July 1981, the President's Commission for the Study of Ethical Problems in Medicine endorsed the total brain death concept. The Commission proposes that a model statute be adopted in every jurisdiction which reads, 'An individual who has sustained either (1) irreversible cessation of circulatory and respiratory functions, or (2) irreversible cessation of all functions of the entire brain including the brain-stem, is dead.' There are a number of criticisms which can be, and have been, made. One of the most obvious is the statute's resurrection of the idea, first mooted ten years previously in the Kansas statute, the first of its kind, that death can be an either/or state. There are not two types of death, there is only death. Any words which suggest otherwise are to be regretted for the confusion they bring. The second criticism is, as I have said, the inability of the statute to escape the intellectual arm-lock of *total* brain death. The reason for this, however, may lie more in the need for the Commission to strike a compromise with certain sections of the medical profession than any inability to analyse accurately the shortcomings of their proposal.

Once the definitional choice is made, the process of determining its existence is a relatively simple technical exercise. In their report on brain-stem, death, published in the *British Medical Journal* of 13 November 1976, the Royal Colleges laid down a code of practice to be followed in determining the presence of brain-stem death. The procedures are carefully designed to provide for the elimination of conditions which could be mistaken for brain-stem death, especially intoxication of the patient from drugs or alcohol or the presence of hypothermia as the cause of the patient's coma. One procedure which is not called for in the British code of practice is the need to take a tracing of the electrical activity of the higher brain by means of an electroencephalograph. Some criticize this as a weakness in the code, but the criticism is ill conceived. As we have seen, death is to be determined by reference to the destruction of the brain-stem not the higher brain. And electroencephalography is quite simply irrelevant to this exercise, since the presence of electrical activity in the higher brain cannot be associated with consciousness once the brain-stem is destroyed. Perhaps the best explanation for this demand for resort to an EEG, which is also reflected in the American decision to opt for total brain death, is that it puts a machine between the doctor and the decision, which is, after all, a decision of the greatest gravity. This is an understandable desire, even if it is not intellectually defensible.

Although I have described the test for determining brain-stem death as a relatively simple exercise, it is, of course, vital that it be carried out competently by appropriately qualified doctors. Once it has been carried out and death confirmed, all the apparatus of life support can, of course, be removed. This may unnerve some, since the heart of the patient is still beating. Once it is realized that it is the machinery and not the person which is making the heart beat, the problem is resolved. And, in any event, when brain-stem death has occurred, the heart will cease beating within a matter of a few days even if the life-support machinery is not turned off.

Finally, it is right to say that satisfactory as the British code is, both in concept and detail, there is one area in which it ought to be amended. At present, there are no provisions which specify the time after the onset of the patient's coma at which the test should be carried out nor the appropriate intervals of time which should elapse before a further confirmatory test is carried out. There are only recommend-ations. Indeed, there is no requirement that the original diagnosis be confirmed, although the code notes that it is customary to do so and recommends it be done. Clearly, in some cases, there is no need to wait to carry out the test. When a patient is admitted to intensive care who has been all but decapitated in a road accident, there can be little question about the confirmation of brain-stem death. On the other hand there may be circumstances in which the patient's coma may be caused by a variety of factors, including drug intoxication. In such a case it may be decided that a more obvious factor — for example severe head injury — is the cause of the coma, and consequently the possible relevance of the drugs could be overlooked. The difficulty is that drug intoxication can, for a short period, produce an impression of brain-stem death. Too hasty a decision to diagnose brain-stem death may be made. The possibility that the patient's condition could be treated, once the effect of the drug intoxication had disappeared, would be overlooked.

There is in my view a need to revise the code to respond to this possibility, unusual though it may be. Specific provisions must be incorporated into the code setting out the time which should elapse before carrying out the test, so as to establish without doubt the cause of the coma. A confirmatory test is not of course necessary strictly speaking if the first test is properly carried out. Nonetheless a provision requiring a confirmatory test and setting out the time interval which should elapse before it is carried out could be incorporated if it were thought appropriate. Only in this way will the residual doubts of a public not yet fully accustomed to the notion of brain-stem death be allayed and the possibility of occasional misdiagnosis be avoided.

Conclusion

In these chapters I have examined some of the dilemmas of modern medicine as I see them. I have sought to unmask medicine. I do not suggest there is anything sinister underneath. There is something of value for all of us once we dispel some of the myths and fancies. I have suggested that there must be a new relationship between doctor and patient. I have suggested that we must take responsibility for our lives. I have suggested that we must challenge the power which doctors exert over our lives. I have suggested that doctors must be made accountable to us. I have suggested ways of redressing the balance of power. I have suggested ways in which a new partnership based on mutual respect may be forged. I have sought to start the debate. Now you must take over.

Bibliography

PRINCIPAL SOURCES

Doyal, Lesley, with Pennell, Imogen, *The Political Economy of Health*, Pluto Press, 1979.

Draper, Peter, *et al.*, *The NHS in the next 30 years: A new perspective on the health of the British*, Unit for the Study of Health Policy, Department of Community Medicine, Guy's Hospital Medical School, 1978.

Illich, Ivan, *Limits to Medicine*, Penguin, 1977.

Inequalities in Health: Report of a Research Working Group, DHSS, 1980.

McKeown, Thomas, *The Role of Medicine*, Basil Blackwell, 1979.

Miller, Henry, *Medicine and Society*, Oxford University Press, 1973.

Muir Gray, J.A., *Man Against Disease: Preventive Medicine*, Oxford University Press, 1979.

Report of the Royal Commission on the National Health Service, Cmnd. 7615, HMSO, 1979.

Townsend, P., and Davidson, N., *Inequalities in Health*, Penguin, 1982.

Wilson, Michael, *Health is for People*, Darton, Longman & Todd, 1975.

The extensive notes and bibliographies in these works are an invaluable source of further material.

SUPPLEMENTARY READING

In Re B (a minor), [1981] I.W.L.R., 1421.

Black, Douglas, '*Cui bono?*', *British Medical Journal*, 29 October 1977, pp. 1109-14.

Black, D., 'Client-oriented medicine', in *Research and Medical Practice: their interaction*, Ciba Foundation, 1976.

Brenner, M.H., *Estimating The Social Costs of National Economic Policy*, US Government Printing Office, 1976.

Campbell, E.J.M., *et al.*, 'The concept of disease', *British Medical Journal*, 29 September 1979, Vol 2, pp. 757-62.

Cobbs v *Grant* (1972) 104 Cal. Rptr. 505, 502 P. 2d 1.

Cochrane, A.L., *Effectiveness and Efficiency: Random Reflections on Health Services*, London, Nuffield Provincial Hospitals Trust/Oxford University Press, 1972.

Davis, Alan, *Relationships Between Doctors and Patients*, Saxon House reprint, Teakfield, 1978.-

Dubos, René, *The Mirage of Health*, Allen & Unwin, 1970.

Duff, Raymond, 'Guidelines for Deciding Care of Critically Ill or Dying Patients', *Pediatrics*, Vol. 64, No. 1, July 1979.

Duff, Raymond, and Campbell, A.G.M., 'Moral and Ethical Dilemmas in the Special-care Nursery', *New England Journal of Medicine*, Vol. 289, No. 17, 25 October 1973, pp. 890-4.

Duncan, A.S., *et al.* (eds), *Dictionary of Medical Ethics*, Darton, Longman & Todd, 1981.

'Fit for the Future', Report of the Committee on the Child Health Services, Cmnd. 6684, London, HMSO, 1976.

Foucault, Michel, *The Birth of the Clinic*, Tavistock Publications, 1973.

Freund, P. (ed), *Experimentation with Human Subjects*, George Braziller, New York, 1969.

Gaylin, Willard, 'In matters mental or emotional What's Normal?', *New York Times Magazine*, 1 April 1973, pp. 14, 54, 56-57.

Glover, Jonathan, *Causing Deaths and Saving Lives*, Penguin, 1977.

The Handbook of Medical Ethics, British Medical Association, 1980.

Jones, Alun, and Bodmer, Walter F., *Our Future Inheritance: Choice or Chance?*, Oxford University Press, 1974.

Jonsen, A., Siegler, M., and Winslade, W., *Clinical Ethics*, Macmillan, New York, 1981.

Katz, Jay, *Experimentation with Human Beings*, Russell Sage Foundation, New York, 1972.

Lalonde, M., *A New Perspective on the Health of Canadians*, Government of Canada, 1974.

Liacos, Paul, 'Dilemmas of Dying', *Medicolegal News*, Fall 1979, pp. 4-7 and 29.

Lorber, J., 'Selective treatment of myelomeningocele', *Pediatrics*, Vol. 53, No. 3, March 1974, pp. 307-8.

MacIntyre, Alasdair, 'Why is the Search for the Foundations of Ethics so Frustrating?', *The Hastings Center Report*, August 1979.

Parsons, T., 'Health and Society', *British Medical Journal*, 1975, 53, p. 257.

People v *Privitera*, 591 P. 2d, 919 (Cal. 1979).

Pickering, Sir George, *Quest for Excellence in Medical Education*, published for Nuffield Provincial Hospitals Trust by Oxford University Press, 1978.

Powledge, Tabitha, and Fletcher, John, 'Guidelines for the Ethical, Social and Legal Issues in Prenatal Diagnosis', *New England Journal of Medicine*, Vol. 300, pp. 168-72, 25 January 1979.

Powles, J., 'On the Limitations of Modern Medicine', *Science, Medicine and Man*, 1. 1:1.

In re Quinlan, 70 N.J. 10 (1976).

Ramsey, Paul, *The Patient as Person*, Yale University Press, 1970.

Reich, W. (ed.), *Encyclopaedia of Bioethics*, (4 vols), Free Press, New York, 1978.

Reiser, Stanley Joel, Dyck, Arthur J., Curran, William J. (eds), *Ethics in Medicine: Historical Perspectives and Contemporary Concerns*, MIT Press, Cambridge, Massachusetts, 1977.

'The 1980 Reith Lectures — some reactions,' 7, *Journal of Medical Ethics*, 173, December 1981.

Relman, Arnold, 'The Saikewicz Decision: Judges as Physicians', *New England Journal of Medicine*, Vol. 298, No. 9, March 1978, pp. 508-9.

Robertson, John, 'Involuntary Euthanasia of Defective Newborns: A Legal Analysis', *Stanford Law Review*, Vol. 27, January 1975, pp. 213-19.

Robinson, David, *The Process of Becoming Ill*, Routledge & Kegan Paul, 1971.

Rollin, Bernard E., 'On the Nature of Illness', *Man and Medicine*, Vol. 4, No. 3, 1979, pp. 157-72.

Sontag, Susan, *Illness as Metaphor*, Penguin, 1977.

Specialized Futures: Essays in Honour of Sir George Goodber, GCB, published for The Nuffield Provincial Hospitals Trust by the Oxford University Press, 1975.

Superintendent of Belchertown State School v. *Saikewicz*, 370 N.E. 2d 417 (Mass. 1977).

Swinyard, Chester A. (ed), *Decision Making and The Defective Newborn*, Charles C. Thomas, Springfield, Illinois, 1978.

Szasz, Thomas, *The Theology of Medicine*, Oxford University Press, 1979.

Szasz, Thomas, *The Myth of Mental Illness*, Paladin, 1962.

Veatch, Robert, *Death, Dying, and the Biological Revolution*, Yale University Press, 1976.

Whitehouse v. *Jordan*, (1981), 1A11 E.R., 267.

Wildavsky, A., in Knowles, J.H. (ed), *Doing Better and Feeling Worse*, American Acad. of Arts and Sciences, 1977.

Wolstenholme, G.E.W., and O'Connor, M. (eds), *Ethics in Medical Progress, with special reference to transplantation*, CIBA Foundation Symposium, J.A. Churchill, 1966.

Working party of the Newcastle Regional Hospital Board, 'Ethics of Selective Treatment of Spina Bifida', *The Lancet*, 11 January 1975, pp. 85-8.

Each of these works has notes and bibliographies for further reading.

GENERAL READING

These are in addition to the books, papers, notes and bibliographies already referred to. They are organized under headings which are intended to serve merely as guides.

Ethics

(i) General

Bok, Sisela, *Lying: Moral Choice in Public and Private Life*, Pantheon Books, New York, 1978.

Hampshire, Stuart (ed.), *Public and Private Morality*, Cambridge University Press, 1978.

Hare, Richard, *Moral Thinking*, Oxford University Press, 1981.

Putnam, Hilary, *Meaning and the Moral Sciences*, Routledge & Kegan Paul, 1978.

Sen, A., and Williams, B., *Utilitarianism and Beyond*, Cambridge University Press, 1982.

Singer, Peter, *Practical Ethics*, Cambridge University Press, 1979.

Warnock, Mary, *Ethics Since 1900*, Oxford University Press, 1978.

(ii) Medical Ethics

Abernathy, V., (ed), *Frontiers in Medical Ethics: Applications in a Medical Setting*, Ballinger, Massachusetts, 1980.

Alting von Geusau, F.A.M., de Locht, P., Dumas, A., and Hellegers, A., *Biology, Ethics and Society: Questions and Issues*, Prospective International, Brussels, 1979.

Beauchamp, Tom L., and Childress, James F., *Principles of Biomedical Ethics*, Oxford University Press, New York, 1979.

Beecher, Henry, 'Ethics and Clinical Research', *New England Journal of Medicine*, Vol. 274, pp. 1354-60, 1966.

Bok, Sisela, 'The tools of bioethics', in Reiser, Dyck and Curran, *op. cit.*

Campbell, A.V., *Moral Dilemmas in Medicine*, Churchill Livingstone, 1972.

Capron, Alexander, 'Medical Research in Prisons', *The Hastings Center Report*, No. 6, 1973, pp. 4-7.

CIBA Foundation Symposium 16, *Medical Care of Prisoners and Detainees*, Elsevier, *Excerpta Medica*, North-Holland, 1973.

A Conversation With Dr Leon Kass: The Ethical Dimensions of in Vitro Fertilization, American Enterprise Institute for Public Policy Research, Washington, DC, 1979.

Cooper, Theodore. 'The Challenge to the Medical Profession', *New England Journal of Medicine*, Vol. 300, No. 21, pp. 1185-8, 24 May 1979.

Curran, William, and Beecher, Henry, 'Experimentation in Children', *Journal of the American Medical Association*, Vol. 10, No. 1, 6 October 1969, pp. 77-83.

Danielli, James F., 'Industry, Society, and Genetic Engineering', The Hastings Center, Readings of the Institute of Society, Ethics and the Life Sciences, 1972.

Davis, John W., Hoffmaster, Barry, and Shorten, Sarah, *Contemporary Issues in Biomedical Ethics*, The Humana Press, New Jersey, 1978.

Dickens, Bernard M., 'Guidelines on The Use of Human Subjects', Office of

Research Administration, University of Toronto, 1979.

Green, Richard, and Money, John. (eds), *Transsexualism and Sex Reassignment*, Johns Hopkins Press, Baltimore, Maryland, 1969.

Gustafson, James, in Williams, Preston N. (ed), 'Genetic Engineering and the Normative View of the Human', *Ethical Issues in Biology and Medicine*, Schenkman, 1973.

Hodges, Lucy, 'Protest to minister on use of drugs to calm children in home', *The Times*, 28 May 1980.

Lappé, Marc, 'Moral Obligations and the Fallacies of "Genetic Control" ', *Theological Studies*, Vol 33, No. 3, September 1972, pp. 411-27.

Lorber, J., 'Results of Treatment of Myelomeningocele', *Developmental Medicine and Child Neurology*, 1971, 13, pp. 279-303.

Mitchell, Basil, 'Is a moral consensus in medical ethics possible?', 2, *Journal of Medical Ethics*, 18, March 1976.

Neville, Robert, 'Ethical and Philosophical Issues of Behavior Control', presented at the 139th Annual Meeting of the American Association for The Advancement of Science, 27 December 1972.

Pub. Law 93-348. *Title II — Protection of Human Subjects of Biomedical and Behavioral Research*, 12 July 1974, 93rd Congress, H.R. 7724, 88 Stat. 348.

Ramsey, Paul, *Ethics at the Edges of Life*, Yale University Press, 1978.

Ramsey, Paul, *The Ethics of Fetal Research*, Yale University Press, 1975.

Ramsey, Paul, 'Genetic Therapy: A Theologian's Response', in Hamilton, Michael P. (ed), *The New Genetics and the Future of Man*, chapter 8, Eerdmans, 1972.

Research Involving Children, Report and Recommendations, The National Commission for the Protection of Human Subjects of Biomedical and Behavioral Research, US Government Printing Office, 1977.

Ryan, Michael, 'Ethics and the patient with cancer', *British Medical Journal*, 25 August 1979, pp. 480-1.

Sanctity of Life or Quality of Life, Study Paper, Law Reform Commission of Canada, 1979.

Stoller, Robert, J., *Sex and Gender*, Science House, New York, 1968.

Thomas, Lewis, 'The Technology of Medicine', *New England Journal of Medicine*, 285 (1971), 1366.

Thompson, I.E., 'Implications for medical ethics of ethics in general', 2, *Journal of Medical Ethics*, 74, June 1976.

Veatch, Robert, 'Models for ethical medicine in a revolutionary age', *Hastings Center Report*, June 1972.

Veatch, Robert, and Sollitto, Sharmon, 'Human Experimentation — The Ethical Questions Persist', *The Hastings Center Report*, Vol. 3, No. 3, June 1973, pp. 1-3.

Visscher, Maurice B. (ed), *Humanistic Perspectives in Medical Ethics*, Prometheus Books, Buffalo, 1972.

213

(iii) Costs, Benefits and Risks

Bailey, Martin J., *Reducing Risks to Life: Measurements of the Benefits*, American Enterprise Institute for Public Policy Research, Washington, DC, 1980.

Calabresi, Guido, 'The Decision for Accidents: An Approach to Non-Fault Allocation of Costs', *Harvard Law Review*, 1965.

Campbell, A.V., *Medicine, Health and Justice, The Problem of Priorities*, Churchill-Livingstone, 1978.

Card, W.I., and Mooney, G.H., 'What is the monetary value of a human life?', *British Medical Journal*, 24-31 December 1977, Vol. 2, pp. 1627-9.

Comment, 'Considerations in the Regulation of Biological Research', *University of Pennsylvania Law Review*, Vol. 126, 1420-46, 1978.

Ferguson, James R., 'Scientific Inquiry and The First Amendment', *Cornell Law Review*, Vol. 64, 639-65, 1979.

Golding, A.M.B., and Tosey, D., 'The Cost of High Technology Medicine', *The Lancet*, 26 July 1980, pp. 195-7.

'Heart Transplants back in favour, surgeon says', *The Times*, 12 September 1980.

Kay, H.E.M., *et al.*, 'Cost of Bone-Marrow Transplants in Acute Myeloid Leukaemia', *The Lancet*, 17 May 1980, pp. 1067-9.

Knox, Richard A., 'Heart Transplants: To Pay or Not to Pay', *Science*, Vol.209, 1 August 1980, pp. 570-5.

Knox, Richard A., 'Mass. General: No Heart Transplants Here', *Science*, Vol. 209, 1 August 1980, p. 574.

Miller, J., and Yandle, B. (eds), *Benefit-Cost Analyses of Social Regulation*, American Enterprise Institute for Public Policy Research, Washington, DC, 1979.

Morley, David, *The Sensitive Scientist*, SCM Press, 1978.

Powles, R.L., *et al.*, 'The Place of Bone-Marrow Transplantation in Acute Lyelogeneus Leukaemia', *The Lancet*, 17 May 1980, pp. 1047-50.

Ross, Walter S., *The Life/Death Ratio*, Readers Digest Press, New York, 1977.

Sauer, Loie, 'Before Proof of Cancer, "High Risk" Women Opt for Breast Surgery', *New York Times*, 23 September 1980.

Swets, John, *et al.*, 'Assessment of Diagnostic Technologies', *Science*, 24 August 1979, Vol. 205, No. 4407, pp. 753-9.

Woodruff, Professor Sir Michael, *Edwin Stevens: Lectures for the Laity: 'The One and the Many'*, Royal Society of Medicine, 1970.

Wright, Pearce, 'New formula costs cancer deaths', *The Times*, 20 March 1980.

Philosophy of Medicine

Blakemore, Colin, *Mechanics of the Mind*, Cambridge University Press, 1976.

Churchland, Patricia Smith, 'A Perspective on Mind–Brain Research', *The Journal of Philosophy*, Vol. LXXVII, No. 4, April 1980, pp. 185-207.

Comment, 'When is a disease not a disease?', *Science News*, Vol. 118.

Engelhardt, H. Tristam, and Spicker, Stuart F., *Evaluation and Explanation in*

214

the Biomedical Sciences, D. Reidel Publishing Company, Dordrecht, Holland, 1975.

Fletcher, Joseph, 'Indicators of Humanhood: A Tentative Profile of Man', *The Hastings Center Report*, Vol. 2, No. 5, November 1972, pp. 1-4.

Huxley, Andrew, 'Evidence, Clues, and Motive in Science', BA Presidential Address, 139th Annual Meeting of the British Association for the Advancement of Science, 31 August-7 September 1977.

Kraupl Taylor, F., *The Concepts of Illness, Disease and Morbus*, Cambridge University Press, 1979.

Nagel, Thomas, *Mortal Questions*, Cambridge University Press, 1979.

Sennett, Richard, 'Books: The Desire to Know', *The New Yorker*, 16 July 1979, pp. 101-6.

Medical Sociology

Baechler, Jean, *Suicides*, Basil Blackwell, Oxford, 1979.

Cousins, Norman, *Anatomy of An Illness*, W.W. Norton & Co., New York, 1979.

Fabrega, H., *Disease and Social Behaviour*, MIT Press, 1973.

Gerson, E.M., 'Social Science and Medicine', *British Medical Journal*, 1976, 10, p. 219.

Horobin, D., *Medical Hubris. A Reply to Ivan Illich*, Eden Press Inc., 1977.

Jarman, Brian, *Health Care in Inner London*, London Health Planning Consortium, 1981.

Kitwood, Tom, *Disclosures to a Stranger*, Routledge & Kegan Paul, 1980.

Loraine, John A., *Global Signposts to the 21st Century*, Peter Owen, 1979.

MacKenzie, W.J.M., *Power and Responsibility in Health Care*, Nuffield Hospital Trust, 1979.

Renvoize, Jean, *Children in Danger*, Routledge & Kegan Paul, 1974.

Ryan, Michael, *The Organization of Soviet Medical Care*, Basil Blackwell, Oxford, and Martin Robertson, London, 1978.

Schofield, Michael, *The Strange Case of Pot*, Penguin, 1971.

Shennan, Victoria, *Mental Handicap Nursing and Care*, Souvenir Press, 1980.

Stimson, G., and Webb, B., *Going to the Doctor: The Consultation Process in General Practice*, Routledge and Kegan Paul, 1975.

Tiger, Lionel, *Optimism: The Biology of Hope*, Secker & Warburg, 1979.

Titmuss, Richard M., *The Gift Relationship*, Pantheon Books, New York, 1971.

Tuckett, D., *An Introduction to Medical Sociology*, London, Tavistock Publications, 1976.

Medical Law and Legal Theory

Bevan, H.K., *The Law Relating to Children*, Butterworth, 1973.

Chatterton v *Gerson*, [1981] 1 All E.R. 257.

Cook, R.J., and Dickens, B.M., *Abortion Laws in Commonwealth Countries*, World Health Organization, Geneva, 1979.

215

Cripps, Y.M., *Controlling Technology. Genetic Engineering and the Law*, Praeger, 1980.

Curran, William J., and Shapiro, E. Donald, *Law, Medicine, and Forensic Science*, Little, Brown and Co., Boston, 1970.

Current Opinions of the Judicial Council of the AMA — 1982, American Medical Association, 1982.

Dickens, Bernard M., *Medico-Legal Aspects of Family Law*, Butterworth, Toronto, 1979.

Hart, H.L.A., *The Concept of Law*, Oxford University Press, 1961.

King, Joseph, *The Law of Medical Malpractice in a Nutshell*, West Publishing Co., 1977.

Law and the Doctor, The Medical Defence Union, 1975.

The Law Reform Commission, *Human Tissue Transplants,* Report No. 7, Australian Government Publishing Service, Canberra, 1977.

Lloyd, D., *The Idea of Law*, Penguin, 1964.

Lloyd, D., *Introduction to Jurisprudence*, Stevens, 1979.

McClean, J.D., *The Legal Context of Social Work*, Butterworth, 1975.

Meyers, David W., *The Human Body and The Law*, Aldine, Chicago, 1970.

Norman, Alison J., *Rights & Risk*, National Corporation for the Care of Old People, London, 1980.

Ontario Interministerial Committee on Medical Consent, *Options on Medical Consent*, 1979.

Paxman, John, (ed), *Law and Planned Parenthood*, International Planned Parenthood Federation, 1980.

Protection of Life: Sterilization, Working Paper 24, Law Reform Commission of Canada, 1980.

Report of The International Conference on the Legal and Ethical Aspects of Health Care for Children, Ontario, 25-7 October 1979.

'The Right to Refuse Psychoactive Drugs', *The Hastings Center Report*, No. 6, 1973, Institute of Society, Ethics, and the Life Sciences, pp. 8-11.

Scott, Russell, *The Body as Property*, Allen Lane, 1981.

Speller, S.R., *Law of Doctor and Patient*, H.K. Lewis, 1973.

Stetler, C. Joseph, and Moritz, Alan R., *Doctor and Patient and the Law*, C.V. Mosby Company, Saint Louis, Missouri, 1962.

Taylor, N.L., *Doctors and The Law*, Oyez Publishing, 1976.

Twining, William and Miers, David, *How To Do Things With Rules*, Weidenfeld and Nicolson, 1978.

Williams, Glanville, *The Sanctity of Life and the Criminal Law*, Faber & Faber, 1958.

Wood, Clive (ed), *The Influence of Litigation on Medical Practice*, Academic Press, 1977.

Politics of Health

'Assurance on invalidity benefit subject to available resources', *The Times*, 22 May 1980.

Battye, G.C., 'Unemployment and Health', *The Lancet*, 7 April 1979, p. 780.

Brenner, M. Harvey, 'Mortality and the National Economy', *The Lancet*, 15 September 1979, pp. 568-73.

Brenner, M. Harvey, 'Unemployment, Economic Growth, and Mortality', *The Lancet*, 24 March 1979, p. 672.

Brewster Kingman, *Edwin Stevens Lectures for the Laity: 'Health At Any Price?'* Royal Society of Medicine, 1980.

Brown, E. Richard, *Rockefeller Medicine Men*, University of California Press, Berkeley, 1979.

Bunn, Rex, 'Unemployment, Morbidity, and Mortality', *The Lancet*, 28 April 1979, pp. 923-4.

Califano, Joseph, *Governing America*, Simon and Schuster, New York, 1981.

'Child Benefit should be top priority', *The Times*, 29 July 1980.

Colledge, Michael, *Unemployment and Health*, North Tyneside Community Health Council, 1981.

Draper, Peter, 'How Can We Make Progress in Health?', presented at the Annual Meeting of the British Association for the Advancement of Science, 1-5 September 1980.

Draper, P., *et al.*, 'Micro-Processors, Macro Economic Policy, and Public Health', *The Lancet*, Vol. i, p.373, 1979.

Erikkson, Jan, *et al.*, 'Unemployment and Health', *The Lancet*, 2 June 1979, p. 1189.

Fagin, L., *Unemployment and Health in Families*, DHSS, 1981.

Ferriman, Annabel, 'Family man will be more than £3 a week worse off in sickness pay under government proposal', *The Times*, 3 April 1980.

Ferriman, Annabel, 'Leukaemia victims die for lack of facilities', *The Times*, 17 June 1980.

Ferriman, Annabel, 'Minister rebuked on health report', *The Times*, 30 August 1980.

Health and Industrial Growth, CIBA Foundation Symposium, Associated Scientific Publishers, 1975.

Health: Sector Policy Paper, World Bank, 1980.

Healy, Pat, 'Grant cuts affect poor families', *The Times*, 18 June 1980.

Healy, Pat, 'Social Security: the Government goes back to basics', *The Times*, 21 May 1980.

Hebert, Hugh, 'Call for better child care likely to go unheeded', *Guardian*, 29 August 1980.

Hebert, Hugh, 'Care worn', *Guardian*, 29 August 1980.

Homeless and Healthless, City and Hackney Community Health Council, 1978.

Jobling, R.G., 'Unemployment and Health', *The Lancet*, 2 June 1979, p. 1189.

Marchasin, Sidney, 'Laetrile: Out of the Lab, Into the Legislature', *Los*

Angeles Times, 30 March 1980.

Meyer, Jack A., *Health Care Cost Increase*, American Enterprise Institute for Public Policy Research, Washington, DC 1979.

'More young people to pay for dental treatment', *The Times*, 11 June 1980.

Morris, J.N., 'Equalities and Inequalities in Health', *British Medical Journal*, Vol. 281, 11 October 1980, p. 1003.

Morris, J.N., 'Social Inequalities Diminished', *Health Visitor*, Vol. 53, September 1980, reprinted from *The Lancet*, 1979, i, 87-90.

Osman, Arthur, 'Best hospital care for "women least in need" ', *The Times*, 15 April 1980.

'Patients First', Department of Health and Social Security, Welsh Office, Consultative paper on the structure and management of The National Health Service in England and Wales, HMSO, London, 1979.

Privitera, James, 'Out of Jail, Back in the Fight', *Los Angeles Times*, 30 March 1980.

Roper, John, 'Can private medicine help the Health Service out of its present difficulties?', *The Times*, 10 January 1980.

Scott-Samuel, Alex, 'Unemployment and Health', *The Lancet*, 3 March 1979, p. 498.

Townsend, P., *Poverty in Britain*, Penguin, 1979.

'Does Unemployment Kill?', *The Lancet*, 31 March 1979, pp. 708-9.

Unit for the Study of Health Policy, 'Effective Prevention: A Comparative Analysis', a short description of a three-year research project unit for the study of health policy, Department of Community Medicine, Guy's Hospital Medical School, 1980.

Wechster, Henry, Gurin, Joel, and Cahill, George F., *The Horizons of Health*, Harvard University Press, Cambridge, Massachusetts, 1977.

Wildavsky, Aaron, 'Wealthier is Healthier', *Regulation, AEI Journal on Government and Society*, January/February 1980, pp. 10-12 and 55.

Young, Robin, 'Low Paid: Hidden snags leave some worse off', *The Times*, 27 March 1980.

Preventive Medicine/Promotion of Health

Ball, Keith, letter to editor on prevention of coronary heart disease, *The Lancet*, 1 December 1979, p. 1182.

Chemical Industries Association, *Cancer in Modern Mortality*, White Crescent Press, 1978.

Department of Trade, *Personal Factors in Domestic Accidents, Prevention Through Product and Environmental Design*, Consumer Safety Unit, 1980.

Ferriman, Annabel, 'Doctors condemn low tax rises on tobacco and alcohol and propose a ban on public smoking', *The Times*, 9 July 1980.

Ferriman, Annabel, 'Smokers resist change of habit', *The Times*, 10 January 1980.

Gibbs, Frances, 'Screening for early diagnosis', *The Times*, 21 February 1980.

Havighurst, C., and Hackbarth, G., 'Private Cost Containment', *New England Journal of Medicine*, Vol. 300, No.23, pp. 1298-1305.

Howard, J. Keir, 'The Prevention of Occupational Cancer: An ASTMS Policy Document — A Review', CIA Background Paper, 20 June 1980. Association of Scientific Technical and Managerial Staffs, London, 1980.

Jones, R. Russell, 'A problem which won't go away', *The Times*, 28 May 1980.

McLaren, Donald, letter to editor on mortality trends, *The Lancet*, 1 December 1979, p. 1183.

McMichael, John, letter to editor on cholesterol, *The Lancet*, 1 December 1979, pp. 1182-3.

Morris, J.N., 'Are health services important to the people's health?', *British Medical Journal*, 19 January 1980, Vol. 280, pp. 167-8.

'National survey on attitudes to smoking: minister's talks with tobacco industry still proceeding', *The Times*, 10 May 1980.

Osman, Arthur, ' "Too few" women having ante-natal tests', *The Times*, 6 May 1980.

Scottish Health Authorities' Priorities for the Eighties, Scottish Home and Health Department, 1980.

Todd, J.E., *Children's Dental Health in England and Wales, 1973*, Office of Population Censuses and Surveys, Social Survey Division, HMSO, 1975.

Todd, J.E., and Walker, A.M., *Adult Dental Health, Volume 1, England and Wales 1968-1978*, Office of Population Censuses and Surveys, Social Survey Division, HMSO, 1980.

Waldron, H.A., *The Medical Role in Environmental Health*, published for The Nuffield Provincial Hospitals Trust by the Oxford University Press, 1978.

Working Group on Back Pain, DHSS, 1979.

Medical Education

Blum, Alan, 'Who Shall Study Medicine in the 1980's?', *Journal of the American Medical Association*, 22-29 August 1980, Vol. 244, No. 8, pp. 779-80.

Chapman, Carleton, 'On the Definition and Teaching of the Medical Ethic', *New England Journal of Medicine*, Vol. 301, No. 12, 20 September 1979, pp. 630-4.

'Cut med schools 13% and many residencies 20%, U.S. panel urges', *Medical World News*, 29 September 1980, pp. 10-12.

Ferriman, Annabel, 'BMA call for limit on training new doctors', *The Times*, 12 April 1980.

Fletcher, C., *Talking with Patients*, Nuffield Provincial Hospital Trust, 1980.

Fordham, Christopher, 'The *Bane Report* Revisited', *Journal of the American Medical Association*, 25 July 1980, Vol. 244, No. 4, pp. 354-7.

'Government Takes Steps to Avert Glut of Doctors', *New York Times*, 2

September 1980, p. C−1.

Parkhouse, J., and McLaughlin, C., 'Career preferences of doctors graduating in 1974', *British Medical Journal*, 2 (1976) 630.

Reproduction and Birth

Ayd, Frank, 'Fetology: Medical and Ethical Implications of Intervention in the Prenatal Period', *Annals of The New York Academy of Sciences*, Vol. 169, 1970, pp. 376-81.

Black, Sir Douglas (Chairman), *Report by the Working Group on Screening for Neural Tube Defects*, DHSS, July 1979.

Bodmer, W.F., and Cavalli-Sforza, L.L., *Genetics, Evolution and Man*, W.H. Freeman & Co., San Francisco, 1976.

Bowman, James E., 'Ethical Issues in Genetic Screening', *New England Journal of Medicine*, Vol. 287, p. 205, 1972.

Dickens, Bernard M. *Abortion and the Law*, MacGibbon & Kee, 1966.

Duncombe, David C., *et al.*, 'Ethical Issues in Genetic Screening', *New England Journal of Medicine*, Vol. 287, p. 204, 1972.

Faith and Science in an Unjust World, World Council of Churches, Geneva, 1980.

Gaylin, Willard, 'Genetic Screening: The Ethics of Knowing', *New England Journal of Medicine*, Vol. 286, pp. 1361-2, 1972.

Hestoff, Charles, and Rindfuss, Ronald, 'Sex Preselection in the United States: Some Implications', *Science*, Vol. 184, 10 May 1974, pp. 633-6.

Lappé, Marc, 'Choosing the Sex of Our Children', *The Hastings Center Report*, Vol. 4, No. 1, February 1974, pp. 1-4.

Lappé, Marc, *et al.*, 'Ethical and Social Issues in Screenings for Genetic Disease', *New England Journal of Medicine*, Vol. 286, pp. 1129-32, 25 May 1972.

Lappé, Marc, 'The Genetic Counselor: Responsible to Whom?', *The Hastings Center Report*, Vol. 1, No. 2, Septembr 1971.

Lappé, Marc, 'Risk-taking for the Unborn', *The Hastings Center Report*, Vol. 2, No. 1, February 1972, pp. 1-3.

' "Live" Abortus Research Raises Hackles of Some, Hopes of Others', *Medical World News*, 5 October 1973, pp. 32, 33, 36.

Memoranda on the Abortion Act 1967 and the Abortion Regulations 1968, The Medical Defence Union, 1968.

Morison, Robert, 'The Human Fetus as Useful Research Material', *The Hastings Center Report*, No. 4, 1973, pp. 8-10.

Murray, Robert F., 'Problems Behind the Promise: Ethical Issues in Mass Genetic Screening', *The Hastings Center Report*, Vol. 2, No. 2, April 1972, pp. 10-13.

Ramsey, Paul, 'Screening: An Ethicist's View', in Hilton, Bruce, *et al.* (eds), *Ethical Issues in Human Genetics*, Plenum Press, 1973.

Reilly, Philip, *Genetics, Law, and Social Policy*, Harvard University Press, 1977.

Snowden, R., and Mitchell, G.D., *The Artificial Family*, George Allen and Unwin, 1981.

Stenchever, Morton, 'An Abuse of Prenatal Diagnosis', *Journal of the American Medical Association*, 24 July 1972, Vol. 221, No. 4, p. 408.

Shaw, Russell, *Abortion on Trial*, Robert Hale & Co., 1969.

Drugs

'Amphetamine Quotas and Medical Freedom', *The Hastings Center Report*, No. 12, 1973, pp. 8-10, Institute of Society, Ethics, and the Life Sciences.

Chowka, Peter, 'The Organised Drugging of America', *The Ecologist*, Vol. 9, Nos 4/5, August 1979, pp. 155-60.

'Doctors urged to cut use of tranquillizers', *The Times*, 28 March 1980.

Duster, Troy, *The Legislation of Morality, Law, Drugs and Moral Judgement*, Collier Macmillan, 1970.

Ferriman, Annabel, 'Better drug guidance demanded for GPs', *The Times*, 3 June 1980.

Grinspoon, Lester, and Singer, Susan, 'Amphetamines in the Treatment of Hyperkinetic Children', *Harvard Educational Review*, Vol. 43, No. 4, November 1973, pp. 515-56.

Halberstam, Michael J., 'Too Many Drugs?', reprinted from *Forum on Medicine*, Vol. 2, No. 3, March 1979, and Vol. 2, No. 4, April 1979, The American Enterprise Institute for Public Policy Research, Washington, DC, 1979.

Klerman, Gerald, *et al.*, 'Controlling Behavior Through Drugs', *The Hastings Center Studies*, Vol. 2, No. 1, January 1974, pp. 65-112.

O'Brien, R. Barry, 'New versions of old drugs help boost Health Service bill', *Daily Telegraph*, 29 November 1979.

O'Brien, R. Barry, 'Wasted spending on brand-names increases health costs by £25m.', *Daily Telegraph*, 27 November 1979.

Reinhold, Robert, 'U.S. Wins Agreement on Warning to Doctors on Use of Tranquilizers', *New York Times*, 11 July 1980.

Wardell, William (ed.), *Controlling the use of Therapeutic Drugs*, American Enterprise Institute Studies in Health Policy, Washington, DC, 1978.

Wardell, William M., and Lasagna, Louis, *Regulation and Drug Development*, American Enterprise Institute for Public Policy Research, Washington, DC, 1975.

Mental Illness

Berthoud, Roger, 'Beyond the headlines — dedicated service to the mentally ill', *The Times*, 2 June 1980.

Breggin, Peter, 'The Return of Lobotomy and Psychosurgery', *Quality of Health Care — Human Experimentation, 1973*, hearings before The Subcommittee on Health of the Committee on Labor and Public Welfare, United States Senate, Ninety-third Congress, First Session, on S.974, S.878, and S.J. Res. 71, 23 February and 6 March 1973, Part Z, pp. 755-77.

Clare, Anthony, *Psychiatry in Dissent*, Tavistock Publications, 1976.

Engelhardt, H. Tristam, and Spicker, Stuart F., *Mental Health: Philosophical Perspectives*, D. Reidel Publishing Company, Dordrecht, Holland, 1978.

Gaylin, Willard, 'On the Borders of Persuasion: A Psychoanalytic Look at Coercion', *Psychiatry*, Vol. 37, pp. 1-9, February 1974.

Gaylin, Willard, 'The Problem of Psychosurgery', manuscript, The Hastings Center Reading 905.

Hodges, Lucy, 'Mental Health Act changes promised', *The Times*, 13 September 1980.

Hodges, Lucy, 'Mental health patients deprived of many freedoms, pressure groups complain', *The Times*, 28 July 1980.

Ingleby, David, 'The Social Construction of Mental Illness', in Treacher, A., and Wright, P. (eds), *The Problems of Medical Knowledge: Towards a Social Constructionism of Medicine*, Edinburgh University Press, 1982.

Ingleby, David (ed.), *Critical Psychiatry*, Penguin, 1981.

Mark, Vernon H., and Ervin, Frank R., *Violence and the Brain*, Harper & Row, New York, 1970.

Mark, Vernon, and Neville, Robert, 'Brain Surgery in Aggressive Epileptics', *Journal of The American Medical Association*, Vol. 226, 1973, pp. 765-72.

'Mental patients' charter for UN', *The Times*, 16 June 1980.

Parry, Hugh, *et al.*, 'National Patterns of Psychotherapeutic Drug Use', *Archives of General Psychiatry*, Vol. 28, June 1973, pp. 769-83.

'Physical Manipulation of The Brain', *The Hastings Center Report*, special supplement, May 1973.

Restak, Richard, *Premeditated Man*, Penguin, 1975.

Rosen, Ismond (ed.), *The Pathology and Treatment of Sexual Deviation*, Oxford University Press, 1964.

Scull, A., *Museums of Madness: The Organisation of Insanity in the Nineteenth Century*, Allen Lane, 1979.

Skultans, Vieda, *Madness and Morals*, Routledge & Kegan Paul, 1975.

Smith, R., *Trial by Medicine*, Edinburgh University Press, 1981.

Szasz, Thomas, *The Myth of Psychotherapy*, Oxford University Press, 1979.

Szasz, Thomas, *Schizophrenia*, Oxford University Press, 1979.

Venables, H.D.S., *A Guide to the Law Affecting Mental Patients*, Butterworth, 1975.

Williams, Thomas A., and Johnson, James H., *Mental Health in the 21st Century*, D.C. Heath & Company, Lexington, Massachusetts, 1979.

Wing, J., *Reasoning about Madness*, Blackwell, 1978.

Death and Dying

Brain Death, determination of: Correspondence, *British Medical Journal*, Vol. 281, 25 October 1980, pp. 910-11, 1139-41.

Capron, Alexander, and Kass, Leon, 'A Statutory Definition of the Standards for Determining Human Death: An Appraisal and a Proposal', *University of Pennsylvania Law Review*, Vol. 121, November 1972, pp. 87-118.

'Declaration on Euthanasia', Catholic Information Services, *Briefing*, 27 June 1980, Vol. 10, No. 23.

Defining Death. Medical, Legal and Ethical Issues in the Determination of Death, President's Commission for the Study of Ethical Problems in Medicine and Biomedical and Behavioral Research, US Government Printing Office, 1981.

'A Definition of Irreversible Coma', Report of the Ad Hoc Committee of The Harvard Medical School to Examine the Definition of Brain Death, *The Journal of The American Medical Association*, 5 August 1968, Vol. 205, pp. 337-40.

'Diagnosis of Brain Death', Statement issued by Conference of Medical Royal Colleges and their Faculties in the UK, *British Medical Journal*, 1976, Vol. 2, pp. 1187-8.

Fries, James F., 'Ageing, Natural Death, and The Compression of Morbidity', *New England Journal of Medicine*, 17 July 1980, pp. 130-5.

Jonas, Hans, 'Against the Stream: Comments on the Definition and Redefinition of Death', *Philosophical Essays: From Ancient Creed to Technological Man*, Prentice-Hall, New Jersey, 1974, pp. 132-40.

Nichols, Peter, 'Vatican says sick need not always be kept alive', *The Times*, 27 June 1980.

Pallis, C., and MacGillivray, B., 'Brain Death and the EEG', letters to the editor, *The Lancet*, 15 November 1980, pp. 1085-6.

'Refinements in Criteria for the Determination of Death: An Appraisal', Report by the Task Force on Death and Dying of the Institute of Society, Ethics and the Life Sciences, *Journal of the American Medical Association*, 3 July 1972, Vol. 221, No. 1, pp. 48-53.

Saunders, Cicely (ed.), *The Management of Terminal Disease*, The Management of Malignant Disease Series, Edward Arnold, 1978.

Veatch, Robert M., 'Brain Death', *The Hastings Center Report*, No. 11, 1972, Institute of Society, Ethics and the Life Sciences, pp. 10-13.

Walsh, Michael J., Moffat, Ronald, Corbishley, Thomas, Harriot, John F.X., and Lakeland, Paul (eds), *The Quality of Death*, Templegate Publishers, Springfield, Illinois, 1975.

Alternative Medicine

Bresler, David E., *Free Yourself From Pain*, Simon and Schuster, New York, 1979.

Law, Donald, *A Guide to Alternative Medicine*, Turnstone Books, 1974.

Worthington, Leonard, 'Unorthodox Healing and The Law', unpublished manuscript.

Consumerism

Cartwright, A., and Anderson, R., *Patients and their Doctors*, Royal College of General Practitioners, 1979.

Cranston, Ross, 'Consumers and the Law', Modern Law Series, Weidenfeld and Nicolson, 1978.

Nader, Ralph, *Unsafe at Any Speed*, Grossman, New York, 1965; adapted, Bantam Books, Toronto, 1973.

Raphael, W., *Patients and their Hospitals*, King Edward's Hospital Fund, 1969.

The Royal Commission on Legal Services, Cmnd. 7648, Final Report, October 1979.

Index